CW01337751

The Sugar & Carb Escape Key

Your Nutritious Blueprint to Losing46lbs (or more) in 6
Months - Without Cravings or Dieting

Sarah Spendiff

For people everywhere who are

both mesmerised and enslaved by food.

May you find your solution within these pages

Reader feedback from advanced copy:

Flipping marvellous - This is a bit weird but even after reading the sample chapters something shifted. Especially around these words... EAT YOUR WAY TO FREEDOM. When truth is told and heard and read and felt. This is the truth to me and I can't wait to start. **Debra Horton**

Well, I have just read the first chapters and it's as if I am reading my own story!! I don't think there is a diet, a gym, a tablet, a system that I haven't tried!! Consistent yo yo! I have just stopped short and talked myself out of trying the injections that are going round!! Every day I wake up, just as you've said, beating myself up about the day before, promising myself I'm not doing that today to a couple of hours later eating toast and marmite! By the slices!! Can't wait to carry on reading - I am buzzing. **Joanna C**

I have...so many friends totally obsessed by their thinking about food all day long, total torture. I note the truths you write about as real, food addiction is real, our attitude to food is manipulated and controlled by our societies reliance on making money through the sale of shit overly processed food. Again, thank you for sharing and I feel you are really touching a nerve and solutions towards oneself. **Cassandra M**

I am two weeks in and can honestly say I am blown away as not only have I lost over half a stone, I feel and look so much better already. I have no cravings for all those foods I used to eat uncontrollably, such as chocolate, biscuits, cakes, pastries and ice-cream. All cravings and obsession Gone! Thank you, Sarah, for sharing your journey with us. I am excited for the coming months. **Fiona Thomas**

It's all really good psychologically for me and physically. I feel healthier, I feel more in control, I feel empowered. I feel more disciplined and that really is my goal, to be more disciplined. Thank you for letting me be one of your prodgies on this wonderful way of eating. **Marie Southport**

The BIG thing is I've completely lost compulsion to gorge on cakes and puddings and I don't snack between meals. Another BIG THING is I enjoy what I eat because the oil, butter and mayo make meals so delicious. I'm a fan and I'm carrying on. **Diane Culverhouse**

Just a few pages in and I'm hooked, I love your writing style, very engaging and I'm excited to continue reading. This is a huge achievement for me to be captivated, at this stage I am usually ready to skip to the programme. **Mel Beeley**

COPYRIGHT

Disclaimer

The information presented in this book is for educational and informational purposes only and is not intended as medical advice. It should not be used to diagnose, treat, or prevent any health condition. Always consult with a qualified healthcare professional before making any changes to your diet, exercise routine, or health regimen. The author and publisher disclaim any liability for any adverse effects resulting from the use or application of the information contained herein.

Launching into the meal plan:

You might be eager to get started right away…

You're not alone, many people want to launch in to losing weight and getting healthier. If that's you, I created the 28-Day Challenge, a structured guide with meal plans and recipes that is getting people incredible results. Find us here www.nuwayoffers.com

* Val M
"I completed Week 1 and lost 6lbs. This made me very happy."
*Siobhan H
Lost 17lbs on completing the 28-Dy Challenge – "I can't say it has been difficult as I love the food."
*Darrly H
I've lost 13.2lbs in less than 3 weeks. I also have more energy, and the clarity of my thinking has improved. I'm also sleeping very well."
*Amanda S
"I've lost 5cm off my waist! And I've lost the desire to eat sweet things."

The 28 Day Challenge includes:

- ➢ Complete meal plans and real food recipes
- ➢ Weekly shopping lists and structure
- ➢ Daily prompts to help you rewire habits
- ➢ A private community of women walking the same path

This is science, structure, and soul — delivered through daily support, nourishing recipes, and a proven path to food freedom.

As a complete reset it takes a deeper dive into mindset, habit forming and emotional eating. Over four powerful weeks you'll rewire the thoughts that sabotage you, learn to eat mindfully and peacefully, discover how sugar and carbs hijack your biology (and how to undo the damage) and finally ingrain planning and cooking skills that other plans do not address.

It's everything I wished I knew decades ago! A proven path to food freedom.

◎ It's a proven path to food freedom.

◎ <u>Join us here</u>

Table of Contents

Introduction
A way out of food obsession
(with a Sugar Addiction Recovery
Plan)

What is the craziest thing you have ever done to lose weight? I thought about going up a mountain once, to live with Buddhist monks for a month because they only eat twice a day and finish eating anything by 12 noon. I thought, after four decades of struggle, what I needed was nonstop meditation and deprivation to fix this faulty wiring that saw me balloon every two years, followed by some drastic diet to restore me to 'factory settings' where I wouldn't be fat anymore.

I never felt like me in my own skin when I was obese. Isn't there a saying, inside every fat woman is a thin one trying to get out? Well, saying or not, I have a solution for you. I lost 46 pounds in six months with this food plan, and being 56-years-old, having struggled and yo-yoed all my life, I personally declare that a miracle.

1

You might be tempted to jump to the food plan and recipes at the back, but I truly recommend you read through the first few short chapters that peel back the layers of the food industry and the health industry - which has contributed to (but not caused) your difficulty, and why this "Food Plan" – not diet – is different.

Now, you might be wondering HOW this book is different from the countless others you've tried. I've spent my life looking for a solution to my obsession with food, weight and diets. Nothing worked – until it did. This is my blueprint to walk you through step by step my research and discovery, in order to release you from an obsession with food and weight.

Here you will learn how you can eat chicken with crispy skin, pork with crackling, have butter on your veg and mayonnaise on your salad and still lose weight rapidly. Why? Because I'll illustrate how you have been deceived by the food industry (and why fat-free food makes you fat) and likely have been deceived by doctors and nutritionists too and how diets set you up to fail. If you are willing to follow the plan outlined on these pages, you'll discover how to lose considerable weight astonishingly fast, and keep it off, without the need for exercising. If this is of interest to you, read on.

Chapter 1

A Lifelong Solution to Weight Gain, Cravings & Carb Addiction

Have you ever felt like you're on a never-ending merry-go-round with food and weight? You try one diet after another, each time believing it might be the solution, only to find yourself right back where you started—or worse off with weight gain and feeling defeated and disheartened. Me too! Many of us have fallen prey to the promises of the diet industry, or the new guru on the block, or a revolutionary new exercise plan, new app, new this new that. If you've ever found yourself in this cycle, I understand your frustration.

I followed diets for most of my adult life. I spent money privately on dieticians, who didn't understand what was wrong with me, and joined diet clubs and /or gyms where I paid a fee to be told I'd gained weight compared to last week!! I've tried every diet under the sun, all the diet books, clubs and programmes you care to mention, but none dealt with, nor understood, my underlying issue. Might this be the case for you?

But there is hope here. More than that, I offer you a roadmap to find freedom from the hold food has over you. If you follow the principles outlined here, you will achieve the figure and freedom you yearn for and deserve. I didn't invent this approach, it's been used for decades, but shrouded in secrecy and prohibited from being shared widely by some arbitrary 'rules' (or traditions). I lost more than three stone (46lbs) in six months, without more strenuous exercise than weekly yoga, and have kept it off to be the healthy weight I was born to be.

Imagine what it would feel like to eat healthily and heartily, without constant worry of gaining weight. What if you could enjoy your meals: crispy chicken skin, pork and crackling, butter on veg, mayonnaise and fruit smothered in full fat Greek yoghurt, without the constant worry of gaining weight. What if you could enjoy your meals, without feeling deprived. This book is designed to help you achieve just that.

Freedom! As the late great George Michael cried

I'm not a nutritionist, or a medical professional of any kind! I just want to make that perfectly clear right from the get-go. What I am is a sugar and carb addict who has had a lifelong battle with weight and food. Gaining and losing weight every few years. If that sounds familiar, stick around—you're in the right place.

I believed the common advice—eat in moderation, choose "healthy" foods, and balance it out with exercise. This is what the new buzz term for the 2020s "calorie deficit" would have us believe. I sometimes shed a few pounds or kilos, but in the end the weight always returned (with interest) and the cravings for the foods that are so hard to give up never truly left. I blamed myself for years, assuming I lacked willpower, that I'm greedy, or just plain useless! But what I've since discovered might surprise you—it isn't about our willpower at all.

I put it to you that the diet industry and the medical industry advice is at best unhelpful, and at worst potentially harmful, for a certain cohort of people. Despite our best efforts, the yo-yo cycle continued, trapping us in a never-ending struggle with food and weight. And if you are identifying with my story, and are still reading this, then you may be in this cohort.

Waifs, Strays and the Whole-Media-Thing

My story is my own, and unique, but the solution I found is one that will work for everyone. Born in the sixties and growing up in the era of Twiggy and with waifs like Kate Moss constantly in the media, I always felt fat, even when I wasn't. I went on my first diet at the age of 12, eating very little and dropping pounds easily. It was the first and only 'diet' that ever worked for me…temporarily.

I didn't realize I was stepping onto the yo-yo diet industry's treadmill, where I would languish for decades, generally wrecking my metabolism—weight up, weight down, though more usually just up. I joined diet clubs and I've been exercising like a lunatic on and off since the 1990s, regularly starving myself. I was desperately seeking a lasting solution and swung between severely restricting calories and then bombarding my deprived body with massive amounts of food.

This back-and-forth left me feeling hopeless. I was consumed with thoughts of weight and diets. I lived in a constant state of mental obsession with food, especially sweet foods and carbs; in trying to deny myself, I ended up miserable, and then powerless over the next binge. It was exhausting, both physically and emotionally, to keep starting over and failing again.

A fundamentally new (for you) approach

If you identify with some of this and are ready to get off this merry-go-round, I have something different to offer: a way to break free of your prison, the noise in your head, the one step forward, two steps back nature of weight issues. What I'm going to share is a Food Recovery Programme. This programme promotes sustainable, long-term change that doesn't rely on costly supplements or restrictive dieting, weigh-ins at a weekly club, or even joining a gym. There are no meal replacement packs, no calorie counting, and no starving yourself; it's not a gimmick or a quick fix.

It's just real food and a straightforward plan to help you drop the weight and keep it off—for good. And it is about more than just losing weight. It's about breaking free from the constant battle with food and weight that so many of us have faced for years. That need to snack and think about food all day long.

I know this approach works because it worked for me and a large group of other people, some with hundreds of pounds to lose—even though it's a little-known way forward. I've lost all the excess weight, and for the first time in my life, it hasn't crept back on. My weight has been stable longer than ever before, and it all started with this plan, allowing me to go about my day without the need or desire for constant snacking or thinking about food.

What we can learn from Addicts

So, what do I know about all this huh? What can I share with you that isn't already in the public domain? Just my own experience of how I busted out of this cycle. I've spent 20 plus years in 12-step programmes for food issues. There are several, and they all differ slightly, but they all derived from Overeaters Anonymous (OA) originally, just as OA itself is derived from Alcoholics Anonymous (AA). AA has helped millions globally recover from "a seemingly hopeless state of mind and body," – i.e. alcohol addiction.

Does it then follow that OA would do the same for food addicts. The answer to that is long and complicated, and outside the scope of this work. Suffice to say, I learnt a lot from all the different food fellowships I attended over 20 years - not least what a food plan is, the addictive nature of food, and how sugar is added to food, hiding in plain sight. It helped, but didn't address my underlying problem. You see, what those food programmes, diet plans, or government advice could not give me, was peace of mind around food. I craved, I obsessed, I yearned, and I mourned food.

I won't go through all the food fellowships and diets I tried as this isn't a book entirely about my journey. It is much more about what I learnt and how I found my way out that I want to share with you. So, I will move on. Suffice to say, it was November 2021, I'm 55 years old at the time and had long since given up on finding a solution to my weight. I had stopped weighing myself once I hit 14 stone (196 pounds) but I'm pretty sure I was way over 200 pounds. I was eating family size bars of chocolate. I ached like a woman 20 years older than I was. I was miserable, I lacked any motivation to do anything, and I looked dreadful, living in tracksuits and huge shirts. I was all out of options. Well, it's darkest before dawn is it not?

Because then I came across little-known food plan that freed me within a few days. It was incredible how well and how quickly it worked. Yes, the weight dropped off which is what we want I know, but I think the freedom is what I value the most. Where once I used to grab the chips from my husband's plate or look on sadly when family and friends indulged their sweet tooth, food no longer has that hold over me, at all. I honestly didn't realise quite how much of my mental faculties were taken up with thinking about, desiring, or craving certain foods and to be free from that is just priceless for me.

If you ever thought that achieving your ideal body weight was an elusive dream, always out of reach, I'm here to tell you that it doesn't have to be that way. This isn't just another diet; it's a food programme—a structured approach to recovery from the madness of dieting. With no calorie counting, protein shakes and weekend treats that trigger the whole cycle again and again.

Following this plan means you'll eat three meals a day, you'll eat abundantly, and you'll avoid foods that are troublesome. You'll find you can go from breakfast to lunch, lunch to dinner without repeated trips to the fridge. You'll likely not think about food at all between meals. Too good to be true? Try it and see. Try it religiously for one week and if you're ready to finally find freedom, you'll find it. I offer you a way out of the madness. It is plan for life that you can take anywhere, that will give you a new lease of life.

Chapter 2

Wait! What if you are Addicted to Sugar & Carbs?

Food is Cunning, Powerful, Baffling

The word addict can sound alarming, but might you see yourself as 'carb sensitive' a problem eater' or even 'insulin disordered'. If you feel you qualify as any of these, this book is for you. I once heard a foodie describe how she became mesmerized by a breadbasket placed in the centre of the table. She couldn't concentrate on the conversation until she'd grabbed a roll, slathered it in butter, and taken a bite. I relate deeply. Food has an unparalleled ability to hijack focus. It's sad, yes, but for those of us with food issues, it's the truth. Sure, skinny people can be screwed up too—they just don't treat food as their solution. And if you're sitting there thinking, lucky them, then congratulations, you're in exactly the right place.

Because this chapter is about the hard truths: what addiction really means, why it keeps some people stuck, and why, if you're obese, you could be dealing with a powerful, deeply entrenched addiction. But then again, this food programme will work for anyone who wants to clean house where their eating habits are concerned. The 'why' of following this plan is unimportant. The result will be the same – lose weight – no cravings – no need to exercise – eat well.

Denial is not a river in Egypt

But for some denial is a real thing. How do you know you have it? Well, that's the million pound question. I remember sitting across from a friend in a café decades ago. She was a big girl; huge, really. I was telling her about my new experience of tackling sugar addiction. She was munching on a chocolate bar at the time, telling me she didn't have a problem with sugar.

I have a relative (or two) who are very overweight, wanting to be slimmer, munching carbs daily and telling me they have this under control. I've seen these same family members skip meals altogether in order to go directly to the dessert. I know the signs. Because I lived them too. I've had many rock bottoms with food, going through phases where I barely ate anything savoury at all, living just on ice cream and chocolate, then grappling back some control, sometimes for long periods of time. The sad truth is, no one can tell anyone else they are a food addict, (or an addict of any kind) it needs to be self-diagnosed. But having said that, this is a way of eating that will work for anyone. You could try it for a little while or forever. The choice is yours. If, however, you have any specific health related illness that could be affected by what you eat, you need to check with your doctor before changing your food regime.

What the Science says.

"Food addiction is a real thing. It's not a metaphor; it's a biological fact. Studies show your brain lights up with sugar just like it does with heroin."

Research indicates that sugar can be as addictive as cocaine. When consumed, sugar triggers the release of dopamine, a neurotransmitter associated with feelings of pleasure and reward. This release mirrors the neurochemical reactions seen in drug addiction and over time these cravings can escalate, making it increasingly difficult to resist sugary foods. Studies on both humans and animals have demonstrated that excessive sugar intake can lead to addictive behaviours, including bingeing, cravings, and withdrawal symptoms.

For instance, a review published *in British Journal of Sports Medicine* notes the similarities between sugar and drugs in terms of their effects on the brain's reward system. We'll explore how sugar is piled high in modern diets, not just in sweet things but in many low-fat items and tons of everyday savoury dishes too. Look at the ingredients on packets of most bacon, bread and even sausages, and you'll find sugar, often under another name (dextrose, glucose, maltose, etc…) it's sugar, nevertheless. Other foods mimic sugar too, such as refined carbs, cereals, juices etc… they all apply equally here.

Man, that mouse is fck'd up

In one study 43 cocaine-addicted laboratory rats were given a choice between cocaine or sugar water over a 15-day period. Forty out of the 43 chose the sugar water. Sadly, but unsurprisingly, mice showed withdrawal from both when they were taken away. Critics will argue (probably rightly) that studies done on rats show what happens to rats, not necessarily what happens to humans. But you don't need to go to medical school to work out when you have a problem with sugar. Although in my experience most people who have a problem with sugar need help figuring out what to do about it.

While many studies, scientists and doctors warn the consumer off sugar and refined carbs, we all know some people (perhaps many people) who can eat these foods safely and moderately. Not everyone is addicted to carbs and sugar. It's a fact, some people can eat these things safely. I'm married to one such person.

When food is placed on the table in front of him, it doesn't suck his focus; when he is eating, he stops when he is full and has had enough, no matter how much he enjoys the meal; he usually eats two biscuits a night, never more (I find this quite irritating!) and he often refuses dessert because he doesn't want one. That kills me too, and generally, if he wants to lose a few pounds he'll tweak his eating habits and then readjust them again, without any difficulty. As a food addict myself, it is his most annoying trait!

But it holds up a mirror to my own struggles. His sympathetic look when I struggle to stay away from the foods that harm me and then beat myself up afterwards. You know that merry-go-round about sugar and carbs that goes on inside your head. He has been on that carousel with me. For the last 20 years in particular, my weight has ballooned by up to 30 pounds a year, only to find me desperate enough to do something drastic to get it back down again. I can't tell you the misery. Until recently I had in my wardrobe all my fat clothes, all size 18s and my virtually unworn, size 10s and 12s.

But I don't diet any more, or count calories, I eat well, and I've been the same size now for years. So, if you really, truthfully have had enough, are ready to change and are prepared to embrace a new way of eating, this plan is for you. That said, you can also use this food plan to drop a few pounds fast, without feeling deprived. I don't want to minimize food addiction, or make light of it, but truthfully, this will work for you if you are not an addict and just want some quick results and time off from some toxic food. My hope is you will feel so well and healthy and happy on it that you'll stick with it.

Eating feelings is nonsense – here's why

As I've already told you, I have great experience at failing in 12-step food programmes. I've tried many, although I expect there are more I could try. All are slightly different and range from not offering any guidance about what you eat at all, to being very regimented to an eighth of an ounce. They definitely work for some, but not for most to be honest in the long term. And anyone who has regularly attended these meetings will attest to the swing door nature of food fellowships.

I'm not going to discourage anyone from attending a food fellowship and finding recovery. You'll learn some good stuff and find a community of people who will support you and with whom you'll have a lot in common. By all means, go, they are free and open to anyone. What I am saying is that without getting the food right in the first place – they won't work for you.

I know because of all the relapses into food I had - despite 'working the programme' and (quite costly to be fair) therapists. It didn't make a jot of difference when it came to caving in to cravings. But when I tried this food plan, within the first 24-hours, the cravings subsided, and they haven't returned. You can head to any 12-step food fellowship, but if you are a serial relapser, or just not a joiner, you can follow this food plan, and I guarantee it will help you.

Food as powerful as drugs

Maybe you believe food has become a coping mechanism for you? Stress, loneliness, boredom are emotions that can drive people to eat, and the food industry knows exactly how to exploit that. Sugary, high-carb snacks are marketed as comforting, indulgent, satisfying. Dr David Kessler, United States Commissioner of Food and Drugs (1990-1997) in the *Fed Up* documentary says, "Processed food is much more powerful than we ever realised. For decades we had the science to show that drugs of abuse can hijack the neural circuits to keep you coming back for more and more. Now we have the science that shows that you can make food highly palatable and that keeps us coming back for more and more and more."

The hard truth is that maybe you are an emotional eater, maybe you don't feel good enough, or loved enough. Maybe food and figure are all tied up with self-esteem, peer pressure, stress, or wanting to attract the right mate. Maybe it's stored trauma that drives you to swallow down food to calm yourself. There are countless reasons for compulsive eating, addictive eating, binging, purging and starving yourself. And you can spend a lifetime on the theory and spend a fortune of therapy, but until you take away the 'triggering' substance, i.e sugar and other foods that behave like sugar, nothing will change.

My name is {your name} and I 'might' be a food addict.

I put it you, you who does not wish to admit defeat, who still thinks scones, and jam and toast and biscuits are your friend: it is time to surrender the battle with food and weight. Surrender to win, resign from the debate. Eat well from the trough of abundant food and have the body and the freedom you were born to enjoy. I'm really not here to convince anyone they are a food addict. Sure, I was 20 years in and out of 12 step food fellowships looking for my solution. But until I eliminated all sugar, grains and starch from my body, nothing was going to work. Perhaps it's the same for you.

Surrender to win

The Alcoholics Anonymous book called *Twelve Steps and Twelve Traditions* opens with Step One and states, *"Who cares to admit complete defeat? Practically no one, of course. Every natural instinct cries out against the idea of personal powerlessness."* It is an accepted tenant among recovering alcoholics that the most profound paradox of recovery is that to beat alcohol you must first surrender. The alcoholic cannot beat alcohol, and so surrenders, and is then able regain control over their lives. This leads to a new freedom and a new happiness.

Therefore, I am speaking to you directly, not the general population; not the person who can eat carbs without huge consequences, gaining a few pounds only, then losing a few when they make a conscious decision to. I'm not speaking to them; I am speaking to you. You who wake up in the morning thinking about food. The person who is still beating themselves up for what they ate yesterday, planning on not doing that again today, then hitting the f@ck it button and eating that carb anyways, and starting the whole darn cycle over again. This is for you, and it might not make for easy reading, but it is life changing, I promise you, stay with me…I got you.

22

I've been eating my feelings all my life!! Food as a reward, food as comfort, food as anything but essential nutrition. Even when restricting, I wasn't normal around food. But after reading all the books, using the apps, having therapy, counselling, dieting, exercising, the end result was the same. It didn't stop me eating the very foods that were making me fat, even though being fat was intolerable to me. So, what was this insane behaviour and how did I change it?

The fact is, breaking free from compulsive eating isn't easy. It requires a willingness to make tough decisions—like cutting out certain foods entirely. Moderation? It's a lovely idea, but for some of us, it's a trap. This means reshaping how you view food. You're not giving up pleasure—you're reclaiming your-self, your life, you're breaking free. Some foods aren't treats - they're chains.

To Conclude:

Food addiction is real. It's powerful, insidious, and deeply-rooted. But it's not unbeatable. If you're ready to break the cycle, you're in the right place. Together, we'll uncover the path to lasting freedom. You need not stare down the barrel of obesity and its related health problems, if you don't want to.

The first step is understanding why you're stuck— the traps of sugar, grains and starch and the flawed advice we've all been fed. In the following chapter we'll explore the diet and health industry's duplicity in this. Following on I'll explain how a food plan works and how to eat your way to freedom. Stay with me—your breakthrough is coming…

Is this for you?

- Have you tried to count calories or count points unsuccessfully?
- Have you ever considered having surgery to help you control your weight?
- Have you had to have treatment or medications to deal with the negative effects of your eating?
- Do you find yourself obsessing over certain foods?
- Do you make up your mind you will eat one way, then in reality eat the foods you know will be counter to your objectives?
- Do you find it difficult to maintain your weight, it is either going up or going down, but rarely stays within the ideal range for long?

- Do you feel like you have tried every diet, app, gadget or book to control your eating to no lasting success?

- Do you have fat days and thin days close together, despite the impossibility of gaining or losing noticeable amounts of weight in a few days? Feeling fat when you haven't changed size is a typical symptom of a person with disordered eating. We call it having a fat head. Also known as having broken eyes (because we do not see ourselves or our food portions accurately) or body dysmorphia.

- If you answered yes to more than one of the questions above, you may be suffering from an eating disorder. I have a solution for you in the next chapter.

Chapter 3

How Official Nutrition Advice Got It So Wrong

For decades, mainstream dietary guidelines—NHS advice included—have pushed carbohydrates as essential for a balanced diet and healthy weight. We were told to stock up on complex carbs like bread, pasta, and rice for "sustainable energy" and to "keep hunger at bay." But for many, especially carb-sensitive individuals (aka people prone to weight gain), this is the worst advice.

You may remember being shown the food pyramid at school in the 1980s which highlighted carbohydrates as the foundation of our diet with tiny amounts of fat at the top? Both the UK and the USA advocated for high carb diets, with the US publishing the first Dietary Guidelines for Americans in 1980 which suggested people should obtain 55-60 percent of their daily calories from carbohydrates.

This advice generally continued in the UK too, when in 1994 the UK Department of Health introduced The

Balance of Good Health, a pretty picture of a segmented plate, which became *The Eatwell Plate* in 2007, and then morphed into *The Eatwell Guide* in 2016. All these have undergone small cosmetic changes, but the advice remains largely the same: a high-carb, low-fat diet with calorie counting (daily 2,000 for women, 2,500 for men) as the golden rule.

Balanced or biased advice?

Where does this advice and guidance come from? To answer that, we need to look back to the McGovern report, published in the US in 1977. It was commissioned by the Senate Select Committee on Nutrition and Human Needs and headed by Senator George McGovern and issued the first warning against diets rich in sugar, carbohydrates and fatty meats.

However, the food industry was outraged about this, and united in rejecting the report and its recommendations on reducing consumption. They demanded a rewrite, and lobbyists got heavily involved, utilizing all the political clout and connection they could. McGovern himself went on the record to warn of this new power of lobbyists to change government policy, but to no avail. The dietary guidelines were revised, and the words "reduced intake" were removed from the report for good. Instead, the report encouraged people to buy more products with less fat.

All this achieved was to spark a whole new food industry at the start of the 1980s in food with the words LOW FAT blazoned across them. This new health craze took every food item imaginable and reengineered it to be low in fat. With the fat removed, these foods tasted terrible. What to do about that? Well, Sugar.

The food industry added sugar to make it worth eating. Some foods had a 50% reduction in fat… but double the sugar content. The end result in the Unites States was that between 1977 and 2000 Americans doubled their intake of sugar. Unsurprisingly then perhaps, in the USA the obesity rate more than doubled from 15 percent in 1980 to over 30 percent by 2000. Along with this rise in obesity came a sharp increase in Type 2 Diabetes.

The Massive Rise in waistlines

The Low-Fat craze hit the UK too with the end result being that between 1980 and 1991 the adult obesity rate doubled from 6 percent to 12 percent. Over this period the UK Government promoted dietary advice that recommended a reduction in fat and pushed the consumption of carbohydrates, suggesting over 50 percent of your intake be carbs.

This significant shift in dietary recommendations set the stage for the rise of low-fat, high-carb diets in the decades to come. Could this be attributed to the increase in sugar and carb consumption and the resulting insulin resistance? This in turn has led people to consume more sugars, processed foods, and unhealthy snacks.

The World Health Organisation (WHO) publishes BMI statistics for the UK beginning in 1966. For decades obesity levels were remarkably constant, as they have been for millennia. But from the 1980s onwards we start see a dramatic rise from 2-3 percent in the 1970's to 27.6 percent for both men and women in 2022. And these figures tally with the UK's own NHS data. In 2021, NHS Digital reported that nearly three-quarters of UK adults aged 45-74 are overweight or obese. Three-quarters! We are supposedly a nation with cutting-edge health technology and knowledge, yet here we are!

Clearly, something isn't working. What changed for UK and US populations in the 1970s and early 80s? Could it be the result of the war on saturated fat, the increased in sugar laden, low-fat foods to hit supermarkets, and the carb-heavy dietary recommendations?

Still the UK government is focused heavily on replacing fats with carbohydrates such as bread, rice, and pasta, which are championed as the foundation of a healthy diet. The most recent government report (2015) Published for Public Health England states: "...the dietary reference value for carbohydrates be maintained at a population average of approximately 50 percent of total dietary energy intake and that the dietary reference value for dietary fibre for adults should be increased to 30g/day." We are now in the situation where two thirds of UK citizens are overweight or obese.

It is hard to prove cause and effect, but this works both ways as those affected by concerns about saturated fat argue there is no undisputed evidence it causes harm.

An article by the USA's Nutrition Coalition, states: "The idea that saturated fats cause heart disease, called the diet-heart hypothesis, was introduced in the 1950s, based on weak, associational evidence. Subsequent clinical trials attempting to substantiate this hypothesis could never establish a causal link."

Food Industry Lobbyist

The power and input of the food industry has been clearly documented in both the UK and US when it comes to issuing dietary guidelines. Dr Zoe Harcombe Ph.D. hits out at the UK government's guidance in her published paper *"Designed by the food industry for wealth, not health: the 'Eatwell Guide'"*.

"Arguably, the high-carb, low-fat diet has been tested on entire populations," says Dr Harcombe, reflecting on her research. "In 1972, only 2.7 percent of men and women in the UK were obese. By 1999, 22.6 percent of men and 25.8 percent of women were obese. That's a nearly 10-fold increase. The overweight population ballooned too, from 23 percent of men and 13.9 percent of women to 49.2 percent and 36.3 percent, respectively."

Is it a coincidence that diabetes followed a similar pattern? In 1980, around 1.42 percent of the population had the disease. By 2015, this rate had soared to 6.1 percent. A causal connection between the introduction of these dietary guidelines and the subsequent rise in obesity and diabetes would seem undeniable.

As Harcombe points out, "the greatest flaw of modern public health advice is its failure to promote real food." With the food industry heavily involved in crafting these guidelines, how could we expect the message to be anything other than flawed?

Clear evidence of this is on record. For example, in 2002 the WHO put together a document known as TRS916 in which they reported that sugar is a major, if not THE cause, of chronic metabolic disease and obesity. The WHO, whose remit is to set global health standards, wanted to restrict sugar intake to no more than 10 percent of daily calories, as recommended by scientists.

But the sugar industry pushed back big time. Tommy Thompson, the U.S. Secretary of Health and Human Services at this time, was asked to stop the report from being published. The Bush administration said the report was 'too tough on the food industry'.

Notwithstanding the fact that the Bush administration received millions in funding from the sugar industry, with sugar baron Jose 'Pepe' Fanjul, head of Florida Crystals, raising at least $100,000 for Bush's presidential re-election campaign.

Lobbyists particularly opposed a recommendation that just 10 percent of people's energy intake should come from added sugar, recommending a x2.5 increase to 25 percent. The government argued that there is little robust evidence to show that drinking sugary drinks or eating too much sugar is a direct cause of obesity and threatened to withhold hundreds of millions of dollars ear marked as the US contribution to the WHO if they published this document.

This resulted in the sugar recommendations being deleted from most WHO documents, up until this day. Incredibly, now, if you look at any food label, you will see that fat, protein and so on, has the daily recommended intake percentage listed. But look at where sugar is listed. Frequently you will see the percentage of recommended daily sugar intake is absent.

The incredible price our kids are paying

Sadly between 1990 and 2000 obesity rates amongst teenagers in the UK trebled to 16 percent and the prevalence of obesity in US children doubled and trebled in teenagers to be 19.3 percent in 2024. This means 1 in 5 children and adolescents in the US are considered obese, and tragically, about 25 percent of children aged 2-5 years old in the US are considered obese. The Bush government actually argued that there is no evidence that selling junk food to children makes them overweight and contributes to metabolic diseases.

It is then perhaps unsurprising to learn we are living in the midst of a diabetes epidemic. Worldwide, says Dr Robert Ratnew of the American Diabetes Association there are approximately 350 million people living with diabetes. Furthermore, it is predicted that one in three Americans will be diabetic over the next 25 years. Dr Ratnew has gone on record as saying one in three Medicare dollars and one in 10 total healthcare dollars, is spent on people with diabetes. There is no question this is a major problem.

Lobbyist, Lies and the Impact on Health

The fact is that food industry lobbying has pressured government bodies to adopt dietary recommendations that favour their products. This includes aggressive marketing by the grain industry, which has promoted grains and cereals as healthy staples, regardless of the growing evidence about what excessive carbohydrate consumption does to a person's health. These interests have often overshadowed emerging scientific evidence that challenges the effectiveness of high-carb diets in combating obesity and related health issues.

In a 2016 study in the Journal of the American Medical Association (JAMA) it was revealed how the sugar industry funded research in the 1960s to downplay sugar's role in heart disease. Historical records also show that the grain industry aggressively lobbied for grains to be considered a cornerstone of the diet. This can be seen in our "Eatwell' guidelines as well as the United States Dept Agriculture's Food Pyramid, which prominently places grains as the largest portion of recommended daily intake during the 1990s.

Many organisations advocating for low-fat diets have received substantial funding from food manufacturers who stood to benefit from the promotion of carbohydrate-rich products. For instance, the American Heart Association (AHA) has been linked to major funding from corporations like Procter & Gamble. The financial ties between these health organisations and the food industry raise questions about conflicts of interest and the integrity of the guidelines produced. For example, the combined revenues of the partners and premium sponsors of the American Dietetic Association are $467 billion, these partners are largely food, drink & drug companies.

Where does all this leave us?

Every year, 4 million people worldwide die as a result of being obese or overweight. The WHO warns that obesity is steadily increasing across all age groups in the UK. In 2022, Frontier Economics estimated the annual cost of adult obesity to the UK is at a staggering £54 billion.

The World Economic Forum estimates that obesity could cost economies globally around $1.2 trillion in lost productivity annually, a reality that can strain not only public health systems but also private sector productivity. Halving obesity rates could save around

300,000 Quality Adjusted Life Years (QALYs) each year. I don't know about you, but I'd like to spend my older years as a QALY—in perfect health.

Despite this, NHS UK still advocates that a healthy plate of food is made up 38 percent of potatoes, bread, rice, pasta and other starchy carbohydrate foods. That's over a third of your daily intake. This advice is propagated all through medical organisations and institutions from health clinics, and NHS dieticians, to the private sector surgeries and even to health food shops.

A Grim Future

By 2050 we could be looking at 90 percent of the UK population in overweight or obese categories and Cancer Research UK has reported that 71 percent will be overweight by 2040. Not just middle to old-aged people, but all people. Imagine what that will do to the NHS with the attendant health concerns. I can't get a GP appointment now—what happens when half the country is dealing with diabetes, high cholesterol, hypertension, and mobility issues?

The British Medical Association has reported that funding cuts and increased demand may lead to a rationing of care, further complicating access to necessary treatments for those most in need. A study by the Nuffield Trust suggests that obesity-related conditions could account for more than 50 percent of the NHS budget by 2030 if current trends continue.

With the government recommending we load up on carbohydrates what chance do people have? This is the end result. An unwell population, increased NHS strain (funded by the taxpayer – you and me) but more profit for the food and pharmaceutical industries. I don't want to get into conspiracy theories but if you look at just one drug used to mitigate the results of poor diet, Lipitor, (just this one statin) has an annual sales value of $12 billion. And we know that people with obesity are nearly three times more likely to develop Type 2 Diabetes: obesity accounts for 30–53 percent of new Type 2 diabetes cases. It's a lucrative cycle.

Dr Michael Klaper MD, a doctor, author and founder of the Moving Medicine Forward initiative says, "The message to all the researchers looking into the cause of diabetes, the cause of hypertension, high blood pressure and obesity, I can tell them in three words. It's the food!"

Dying from Excess and Ignorance

Let me qualify that heading please. Overweight people are NOT greedy, and they are NOT lazy and certainly NOT stupid. They (we) have been lied to frankly, mislead, conned and deceived, over and over. I (we) literally at times have not known where to turn to get it right. But we should all question the guidelines that have been handed down and to question if they are in our best interest.

The debate continues, but the damage caused by decades of misleading advice is evident, isn't it? As we think about the obesity crisis, we can see how these early guidelines shaped our eating habits and the broader public health landscape. But… these academic debates are not the point of this book. I want to help you, specifically you, find a way out of your prison. If you've been struggling with the NHS's carb heavy, low-fat recommendations that have been round a long time and feel you're not getting anywhere, I think I can help you.

If we disregard the officialdom recommendations on what foods we should be eating, as many people do, that leaves us with the private sector diet industry, and they're cleaning up where the official advice is failing the population. Trying and failing with one weight-loss method after another, I had resigned myself to just stay failed, as my fat clothes no longer fit, and I couldn't bear to look at myself. But now I have paved a new path toward recovery and lasting health. And I may well have a lasting solution for you too. Read on.

To conclude

- NHS *Eatwell Guide* says carbs are essential for energy and should be a huge part of your plate, despite ever growing obesity levels
- Much of the research and guidelines have been tainted via competing interests and lacks credibility
- Most low-fat food is laden with sugar
- For better metabolic health, fewer cravings, and actual weight loss that sticks, rethink your relationship to fats, low-fat fads and carbohydrates.

Chapter 4

The Diet & Exercise Lie: Why you Can't Outrun Cravings

Up-to-date data from the market research company *Market Data Forecast* estimates that the diet food industry is worth $326 billion in 2024 and is predicted to reach $347.5 billion by 2025. By 2032, the weight loss and diet management market is projected to value $628.37 billion. A staggering number by any measure, and one that covers everything from meal-replacement shakes to weight-loss surgeries.

Yet there are 1.5 billion overweight or obese adults in the world, despite this hugely 'successful' and lucrative business! We know that more and more people are dying of heart disease and diabetes than ever before! Something is not working, and you have to ask yourself, what the heck is going on?

After reading the previous chapters you will understand why I do not entertain any armchair advice from people, even professionals, about what I "should eat". I know what I need to do, and I know it will help you too. But first let's take a quick look at the current diet and exercise rages propagated on your socials and elsewhere.

Drinking Diet Industry Kool-Aid

In the 2000s, a wave of research began to challenge the low-fat, high-carb approach. Studies showed that it was not fat, but refined carbs, particularly sugars, that were contributing most to obesity, insulin resistance, and metabolic disorders. The idea that fat is the enemy of health had started to be challenged. Enter the Atkins *New Diet Revolution,* that turned official advice on its head.

Initially discredited and highly controversial, due to its radically different approach, it was created by Dr. Robert Atkins in the 1970s, but didn't gain traction until 1990s and 2000s. The primary aim was to drastically reduce carbs and increase protein and fat consumption. Other high-protein, low-carb diets followed, as people found significant success, losing weight and improving blood sugar control by reducing their carb intake and increasing their fat intake. Low-carb, high-fat diets remain very popular.

I don't promote any established diet, I tried so many of them and still ended up in despair and weighing over 14 stone, a lot for my 5ft 5in frame. We now know that Atkins himself died overweight, clinically obese in fact, and that he also suffered from heart disease, so while I'm not in any way trashing the premise, I am saying that what I do now is different from typical high-protein, low-carb diets. I drank the Atkins 'Kool-Aid' in my day, I bought his book. I did lose weight, but did not find the freedom from food obsession that I now enjoy. And with one slice of bread, the fat was back.

I also bought *The Dukan Diet* book, a similar high-protein low-carb diet devised by Pierre Dukan. I also tried the *Scarsdale Diet* of course, a high-protein low-carb fad diet created by Herman Tarnower. Similar to the Atkins Diet, it is high in animal protein but restricted to 1,000 calories per day and lasts between seven and fourteen days. The question is, then what? I need a sustainable solution that lasts a lifetime and thank the heavens I've found it.

What about the other end of the spectrum, remember the *F-Plan Diet*? Authored by Audry Eyton in 1982 *the F-Plan Diet* is low in fat and high in fibre and theorises that because fibre fills the stomach it will reduce the desire to overeat! A criticism of the diet is that it can cause constipation and flatulence due to its recommendation of consuming 35–50g of fibre per day. Giving rise to its nickname the "Fart-Plan Diet". Nevertheless, it was translated into sixteen languages and had sold over three million copies by 1985. No doubt making Eyton very wealthy and credited with increasing the sales of bran-based cereals by 30%, wholewheat bread by 10%, wholewheat pasta by 70% and baked beans by 8%. As we've discussed, the diet food industry is big business.

There are very many more diets I've tried, many I'm sure you are familiar with too. I've done the *Cambridge Diet*, (and other incantations of it - Slimfast, Lighter Life etc.) restricting my calorie intake to less than 1000 through 'complete meal shakes'. I find it easier to not eat at all, than to moderate calories, and if you relate to that, then we've a lot to talk about. The shakes work initially but are not sustainable. You probably know that already.

No doubt some diets work for some people, but not those of us who are carb sensitive. Those of us who suffer from an allergy to certain foods. As previously mentioned, an allergy is just an abnormal response. In our case, the response is once we start, we just can't stop, despite the consequences. That is the very definition of an addiction.

While some people can moderate, reduce and so on, unless we 'problem eaters' clean our palettes completely of the troublesome foods, even the smallest amount sets of a sense of craving, yearning for (insert your sugar / carb preference here). This becomes an obsession of the mind, so overpowering it has the ability to get me to put on my coat, get in the car and drive to the shop, simply and purely to indulge this craving. No other substance (since I gave up alcohol) has the power to do that to me. Thankfully I've regained control of myself and my life and follow through with me and you will too, I promise.

The Role of Pharmaceuticals

Duromine. I got it prescribed by a doctor, who suggested I eat half of my usual portions and stay on the pills for no more than three months at a time. I'll never forget those days, and I'm pretty sure I permanently damaged my health with them. They are basically amphetamines, otherwise known as the street drug 'speed'. Sure, not eating while on the drug is easy.

Other side effects were, I cleaned the house from top to bottom, barely slept, and was very anxious.

But the weight goes right back on once you stop taking them, which you must as they have diminishing returns anyway. Having not felt hungry while on them, I was ravenous when I stopped, and exhausted too, doing nothing but sleeping and eating. Incredibly I went on this cycle for months at a time.

Phentermine is one of the most popular weight loss drugs prescribed and is a stimulant too. It carries a risk of dependence and is therefore a 'controlled' drug. It works as an appetite suppressant, loses effectiveness for most people after a time, and many who lost weight on it gain it back.

There is now a lot of hype around Ozempic, a trade name (there are others) of the active ingredient 'GLP-1 agonist'. I haven't tried it and if you want to and can afford to, that's up to you. However, despite only being a relative newcomer on the block, it's gained wide media coverage and therefore popularity. But studies into its use are starting to come to light.

Medical News Today referred to a 2022 study that explored changes in body weight and metabolic risk factors among 1,961 participants one year after treatment. The authors found that stopping taking the pills can cause a person to regain lost weight and that they may also notice increased cravings and blood sugar spikes.

The study stated: "One year after withdrawal of once-weekly subcutaneous semaglutide (the medical name used for the active substance in Ozempic, also known as GLP-1) 2.4 mg and lifestyle intervention, participants regained two-thirds of their prior weight loss, with similar changes in cardiometabolic variables."

The study recommends "ongoing treatment to maintain improvements in weight and health". I find that frightening to think that the only way drugs like Ozempic will help you is if you keep taking them and keep paying the drug companies for them. In conclusion, so-called diet pills are a terrible idea.

NB:A review by the University of Oxford (published in May 2025) looked at 11 studies on both older and newer GLP-1 weight loss drugs. It found that people typically lost around 8kg while using the injections — but within 10 months of stopping, most had regained the weight.

Even those on the newer, more powerful drugs like Wegovy and Mounjaro — who lost an average of 16kg — started regaining weight once treatment stopped. On average, they put back on 9.6kg in just 12 months, which suggests that without ongoing medication, the full amount lost could return within two years.

The Diet Industry's Deceptions

If we're facing facts, the diet industry thrives on creating a cycle of dependency and failure. It perpetuates the myth that weight loss is merely a matter of willpower and discipline. Calories in versus calories out. But this simply isn't true. It won't come as a surprise to anyone that restricting food intake only works in the short term for some, and not at all for others!

Studies show that 80-95% of dieters regain lost weight within 1-5 years, underscoring the cycle of hope and disappointment that many experience. The fleeting success often leads to a renewed struggle with weight, reinforcing negative self-perceptions and contributing to emotional distress.

For example, low-carb plans, though effective initially, often lack the structure necessary for lasting adherence, leading to eventual weight regain. Programme that offer meal replacement shakes promise rapid weight loss through extreme calorie restriction but rarely prepare dieters for the reality of dealing with food long-term. These fleeting successes aren't a bug of the system—they're the feature. After all, a business model that fixes you once and for all, hardly makes good business sense, as there is no repeat custom. And gyms, clubs, meal replacement providers and those that offer shakes, rely on repeat business.

The Issue of insulin

Insulin, the so-called "fat-storage hormone," governs energy storage and usage in our bodies. Honestly, I've got super confused about insulin and how it works in weight gain, weight loss, diabetics, etc... but I've recently had my 'aha!' moment.

I was confused by the 'all calories count mantra' of the food industry. And it is true that all calories will be broken down to make glucose. However, the secret is in how they get broken down and this is where insulin, and indeed insulin resistance comes in. For example,

200 calories of apples will be digested with a shed load of fibre. This slows the process through the digestive tract, turning slowly to energy.

However, 200 calories of apple juice blasts through the system, into the liver which is overloaded with sugar, which it just can't handle or process alone, so it hits up the pancreas to release insulin. The insulin goes about swiftly cleaning the system of excess sugar, turning it directly in to fat. That is what insulin does, it's triggered by excess sugar, and turns that excess sugar to fat. The end.

Below is how the clever books explain it, I think my way is clearer, but here is the techie speak from wiki something: "When we eat refined carbohydrates like sugary snacks, soda or sweets, they convert into glucose, causing a blood sugar spike. The pancreas releases insulin to manage the glucose surge, helping cells absorb it for energy."

Starchy carbs—once touted as the backbone of a healthy diet—cause a metabolic disaster. Foods like cereal, bread, pasta, and rice spike blood sugar levels, as instantly as plain sugar, triggering a cascade of insulin responses. The inevitable crash leaves you hungry, lethargic, miserable and primed to do it again.

This endless eat-spike-crash-crave cycle keeps us hooked. Over time, the body can develop insulin resistance—a condition where cells stop responding effectively to insulin, forcing the pancreas to work ever harder. This dysfunction is a precursor to Type 2 Diabetes and is strongly linked to obesity.

The food industry exploits this hormonal hijack to perfection. Low-fat and diet products, laden with added sugars, spike insulin levels and trigger more cravings. This clever manipulation guarantees we stay dependent, both biologically and financially.

It has helped me to understand this, that not all calories are the same and the way that cravings for sweet things, although making me fat and miserable, kept me going back for more of the same. Was I insane? Einstein's definition of insanity is doing the same thing over and over, expecting a different result. That clearly made me mad.

Insulin and the PCOS connection

A little-known fact is that polycystic ovary syndrome (PCOS) is related to abnormal hormone levels in the body, including high levels of insulin. It means that some women with PCOS are insulin resistant and are at increased risk of becoming overweight, developing Type 2 Diabetes, high blood pressure and high cholesterol!

While we all respond with a spike in insulin as soon as any carbs are consumed, in those with insulin resistance PCOS, this process becomes dysregulated. In these cases, the body produces more insulin than necessary. This excessive insulin can cause blood sugar levels to drop too quickly, leading to hypoglycemia (low blood sugar). The result is intense hunger and cravings for more sugar or carbohydrates to replenish glucose levels, creating a vicious cycle.

Sadly, the brain's reward system also gets involved because carbohydrates can trigger dopamine release, a feel-good neurotransmitter. When insulin levels spike and then crash, the brain craves more sugary foods to restore dopamine levels, reinforcing the cycle of cravingsInsulin resistance is a real problem for many of us who struggle to maintain weight loss and stabilise our blood sugars.

Calories in Calories out debacle

The idea that low-fat diets and more exercise is the solution has been failing for over 50 years. Between 1980 and 2000 fitness club memberships more than doubled across the United States. During that time the obesity rate also doubled and today two thirds of Americans are overweight, despite ever increasingly complex exercise regimes and fad diets. This situation is dire.

Margo Wootan, director of Nutrition Policy, Centre for Science in the Public Interest. "We are not going to exercise our ourselves out of this obesity problem." She says but adds that exercise has many health benefits, "but to burn off just one 20-ounce coke, a child would need to cycle for 75 minutes. Most people just don't have that much time in their day."

A view agreed upon by Gary Taubes, bestselling author of the Diet Delusion, highlights how energy balance propagates a myth that if we match the calories in - to the calories out we will tackle the weight issue, and says this is nonsense. "You eat say 110 bites of food a day, and only burn off 109 of them, you'll be obese in 20 years. Even a Guinness world record holder of counting calories could not do that, nobody can do that."

The message that we have been gobbling up for decades is, 'moderate', have a little of what you like (not too much) and make sure you expunge the calories through a balanced diet and exercise. And for those of us who fail at this time and time again, the message is…you are lazy and lacking in willpower, it's on you, all on you, when in reality…it's the way these foods are processed in your body.

My hope is that by understanding the deceptive nature of the diet industry, the role of lobbyists in government advice, along with the role of sugar and starch in our diets, you can take the first step toward genuine recovery and sustainable health. If this book has spoken to you so far, read on to find your solution.

To conclude

- Between 80%-98% (depending on sources) of people don't lose weight or regain what they lost, only 2% of people maintain a 20lb weight loss

- Robert Atkins - the founding father of high-fat, low-carb dieting was clinically obese when he died according to his released post-mortem
- Zoë Harcombe, author and nutritionist believes that eat less/do more has never worked and will never work
- If the calorie theory were correct, every human would lose 104 lbs every year, with a 1,000 calorie a day deficit (no matter their gender, starting weight etc)
- There are 0 vitamins & minerals in sugar

Chapter 5

How to Eat Your Way to Freedom & Shut Down Sugar Cravings

How it Works

One of the most brilliant things I have ever heard in a 12-step food program is: "How do I know I am food addict? Because I mourn the passing of food."

When I knew I had to give up chocolate, I honestly felt suicidal. And truthfully, when you put down your addictive substances, you will feel some feelings. But it is important to remember; "feelings are not facts" and "this too shall pass". Sometimes it is just about holding on until the feeling has passed. Every single time you respond to a feeling without eating on it, you grow and get stronger. Because we do not JUST stop eating sugar, grains and starch on the food plan, we have a structured plan of eating that I am going to lay out for you below.

This means eating three meals a day, with nothing in between. It is a disciplined way of eating. If you are still here reading this, then you have come so far in acknowledging you have previously suffered with Disordered Eating. This plan is about ordered, conscious eating. Why is this important? Largely because regaining control of yourself, your body and your eating, means not using food as a reward or motivator. Let me explain. I once read Melody Beatty (a well-known 'recovery' writer) explain how a food addict or compulsive over eater (define it as you will) tends to inhale calories and not know they are doing it. That line really struck me, as it was so true for me.

I had emphatically believed that there was no need to include a healthy snack to my food prep - as I never snacked. What rubbish, I grazed constantly. I literally didn't see it until I put the conscious structure in place; three meals, three times a day, nothing in between. It was actually completely liberating, there was now no debate around snacking. You will find with this plan that there is enough delicious food to get you from breakfast to lunch, lunch to dinner. And then do it again the next day. Your blood sugar will stay stable and your brain stays focused on the task at hand – not straying to snacking. It's astonishing how well this works.

57

A Food Plan is Not a Diet!

I adapted this food plan through all I learnt while attending 12-step food fellowships, and these are not diet clubs. They tackle issues that are far more complex around food behaviour, such as compulsive over-eating, bulimia and anorexia. I have directed this food plan specifically to over-eaters like me and we are a complicated co-hort. We not only 'overeat' but most often we eat foods that we know won't help us, but we cannot help ourselves! However, bulimics and anorexics may find this food plan helpful too, and I hope they do try it. But I do not have personal experience of these disorders, and it is my personal experience that informs this work.

The three weighed and measured meals a day, with nothing in between, is the key to your freedom. You will eat well and plenty, often cooking from scratch to avoid processed food with added sugar and grains. I have some handy tips to cut prep time and I spend far fewer hours in the kitchen now than I used to when food was everything to me. You need to allow four hours between each meal, but do not let more than six hours pass before your next meal, as this leaves you vulnerable to making the wrong choices. It is a manner of eating that really works. You can drink unlimited black or herb tea, black coffee and sugar free drinks. One of the reasons we do not drink unlimited hot drinks with milk initially (i.e. during Weight Loss) is because as addicts we look to fill ourselves up with anything, so we measure our milk intake.

There are three phases to the program which are Weight Loss, Management and Lifetime. Initially this will take some getting used to, but if you persevere with all the shopping and chopping you won't look back, and there are always short cuts and handy hacks which we will get in to as well. This food plan - program of recovery if you will – has been adapted over 20 years of trial and error.

Most of the 12-step food fellowships that offer a 'meal plan' do not share them, there are no digital copies, and they are given either verbally or by hard copy. This secretive method of sharing a life-saving food remedy prevents countless people from regaining their health and living peacefully on this planet with food. I don't agree with that and have therefore used my considerable experience with what works, what fails, to bring this amazing food program to as many people who need a way out as possible.

A Word of Caution

Having said that, if you deviate from the plan at all you will either find cravings return (if you eat sugar, grains or starch) which really sucks and the weight loss will stop. Let me explain further. Having adapted this program from 12 step fellowships that never deviate from the food plan, I've incorporated the three stages in order to adapt the program for 'normal living' to ensure a lifetime of freedom from cravings. It has been a great success for me and the countless others who have tried it. But while you are on Weight Loss, you need to stick to the exact measurements and the correct foods, a full list of which is in the appendix.

So, while we exclude specific foods in Weight Loss, some can be reintroduced in management, but be warned, you may find that this is when the weight loss will stop. Also, if you start to adapt the salad and veg portions, likewise this may affect your weight loss. And once you have become more flexible with measurements and variety (which is actively encouraged in Management Phase) please be aware, you are unlikely to be able to put the genie back in the bottle, if you decide later to lose more weight. So, to drive home the point, for weight loss, adhere accurately to the plan. If you do not, you cannot bemoan the result.

However, now is not the time to worry about deviating from the plan, the current focus is on learning this way forward and losing weight the easy way, without cravings, hunger or feeling deprived. Management and Lifetime will be thoroughly explained as we move forward.

Change your eating habits – change your life

- "What do we want"
- "Weight loss"
- When do we want it?"
- "Now"

I'm not trying to be irreverent; body weight challenges are a serious concern and have made many of us miserable for a very long time. I dropped over three stone (46 pounds) in my first six months on this plan to become a slim and healthy 10 stone. One of my friends lost 10lbs in 20 days. How much you lose will depend on your own metabolism, and how much you have to lose, but expect rapid results, which will stay off for life if you follow this food program.

As you now know we eliminate all sugar, grain and starch from our daily food intake for the Weight Loss phase and instead eat a whole range of nutritious real food. All proteins are on the food plan; beef fat, prawns, pork crackling and bacon, cheddar cheese melted over vegetables and smothered in butter are all included. I promise you'll be able to eat delicious, full fat versions of food and providing you stick to the food plan; you will lose weight. A cautionary note though, people will nag, judge and criticize. Let them. You are on a new path to a freedom hitherto unknown and one that has been checked and recommended by health providers and tried and tested on thousands and thousands of people. It's safe, it works and is a huge improvement on what we were eating before.

Setting you up for success

These things will help you:

- **A DIGITAL BATHROOM SCALE**: It is recommended you weigh yourself no more than once a month. Do weigh yourself on Day One and make a note of your weight. But then weigh yourself again on the first of the month, no matter how soon that comes around, and then every first of the month thereafter, making a note of your weight.
- **TUPPERWARE,** food containers, and food bags. This is so helpful for storing food as it is encouraged to cook in batches. It is also so helpful for travelling and eating away from home.
- **A DIGITAL KITCHEN SCALE** and a smaller one for travelling with, plus spare batteries.
- **LITTLE PLASTIC BOTTLES** used for taking creams on holidays. Ideal for oils and dressings when travelling.
- **PLAN YOUR FOOD**. Fail to plan, then plan to fail. I cannot stress this enough. Write out what works for you in terms of proteins, fruits, vegetables and salad, for every meal either the night before or early in the morning. I do a big shop and write up my meal plans for the next four days. Other people do

theirs daily. You'll see what suits you but knowing in advance what you are going to eat, never winging it, but planning it, is #1 key to success.

- **SIMPLICITY:** In the early days you are encouraged to keep it simple. Do not hesitate to eat the same thing if it works for you having shopped and cooked in bulk. The same thing for lunch two days in a row, or two meals in a row is no hardship when it's good food that you like. You will learn new and interesting ways with the food plan as you go along.

- **EAT AT HOME**: Avoid socialising around food in the early days. You will find there are other things to do with friends than eat. In later stages you can go anywhere and do anything, but while we instil a new relationship with food, protect your abstinence above all else.

These things will not help you

- Deviating from the plan.
- Eating out will be difficult at first. Restaurants do not offer large enough portions of the food we do eat, and who knows what they may have added. To set yourself up for success, it is best to avoid eating out in the early days.

- If eating out cannot be avoided, look up the restaurant's menu beforehand so you know what you can order to protect your abstinence.
- Not checking labels for additives, we do not eat. There are up to 60 different names for sugar and sugar derivatives. Be cautious and read the labels. Flour and types of flour are also added to a huge range of food where you wouldn't necessarily expect to find it.
- Do not go more than 6 hours without eating, but if you ate less than four hours ago, you do not need calories. You may have emotional hunger, ride it out.
- Telling people what you are doing. People will criticise and judge. Many will not understand. Don't try to convince anyone of anything, just stick to what works for you.
- Do not get too Hungry, Angry, Lonely or Tired. This is the HALT advice used to guide recovering addicts to look after themselves. Hungry: Is it time for your meal? If not, there is one coming soon. Or you may be thirsty, drink plenty of water. Angry: Feelings such as anger may arise more easily or for no reason. This is to be expected after stuffing down feelings with food for years. Talk to someone about

how you feel, rather than act on it. And finally Tired. This is an easy one, rest. In fact, we say to put yourself in intensive care in the early days. Rest, sleep, relax, watch telly. Happily, this program works even if you do not exercise.

To Conclude:

- In this chapter we have given a broad outline to the food plan as well as insight to the origin of it, developed over 20 years in 12-step food fellowships.
- This chapter also provides a glimpse into the roadmap towards freedom from obsession with food, diets and weight.
- We highlight here how, by adopting a structured and conscious way of eating, you can break free from cravings, guilt and the endless cycle of weight gain with occasional weight loss.
- This food plan is nothing short of miraculous for those who identify as being carb-sensitive, a food addict or for whom traditional diets do not work. In other words, for many of us.
- This is an incredibly powerful way of living and eating, and I'm excited to be joining you on your journey to freedom. In my next chapter I lay out the food plan with meal examples in more detail.

Chapter 6

Astonishingly Fast Weight loss – With Real Food and Big Meals built-in

What and how to eat

To be explicit about what we eat on the Weight Loss phase of this is plan: three weighed and measured meals a day, nothing in between, and no sugar, grain and starch. That might feel hard but try it at least once for 24 to 48 hours. People who do try it love it, and don't look back. Below I outline your food groups, and most importantly, the volume of food you will be eating, because we eat plenty at every meal. You will feel nourished AND satisfied.

The full list of foods we eat are in the appendix, but I outline it below with a few examples in case that is helpful. But do check your choice of fruit, salad and vegetables in the appendix, as we do not eat all of them. Use your digital kitchen scale, and you will weigh out:

- Breakfast: One full portion of Protein + 8oz Fruit + (optional) 2oz milk for tea/ coffee

- Lunch: One full portion of Protein + 8oz Salad + 8oz Vegetables + 1oz Fat
- Dinner: One full portion of Protein + 8oz Salad + 8oz Vegetables + 1oz Fat
- (NB: With each meal you have the option of adding 0.5 oz (15 grams) of seeds

Cook your food however you like, you can follow your own recipe but only add ingredients on the food plan list in the appendix. You can add whatever herbs, spices, fat free / sugar free dressings you like. I use balsamic vinegar on my salad, but it's up to you. You can add mustard and soy sauce (however, if you are having issues, suggest you find the wheat free version of soy sauce, it does exist).

Vegetables can be boiled, grilled, roasted or air fried and you can add a 1tsp of oil for cooking. The same goes for cooking the proteins, cook as you like, and use a little oil if needed. This does not count towards the 1oz of fat you add to your plate.

All measurements are **the cooked weight**; therefore, cook up plenty to ensure you have enough. Batch cook and stick leftovers in the fridge or freeze for later. You will end up with tons of Tupperware, and bits of food and it's all helpful.

A typical lunch might look something like this:

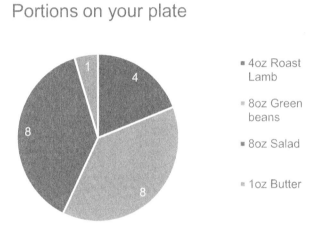

Fig.1 plated portions example

The Food Plan in more detail

Not all Proteins measurements are the same:

Protein	Full portion (Men)	half portion	quarter portion
All meats	4oz (6oz)	2oz	1oz
All fish	4oz (6oz)	2oz	1oz
Milk	16oz (24oz)	8oz	4oz
Yogurt	8oz (12oz)	4oz	2oz
Eggs	2 3	1	N/A
hard cheese (e.g. cheddar, Gauda	2oz (3oz)	1oz	0.5z
White cheese (e.g feta, goats)	3oz (4.5oz)	1.5oz	0.75oz

Edamame + Soya beans	4oz (6oz)	2oz	1oz
Tofu	4oz (6oz)	2oz	1oz
Soybean flour	4oz (6oz)	2oz	1oz
Seeds (Sesame, flaxseed, chia only)	0.5	N/A	N/A

Fig 3: table of portion sizes

Why have I given percentage of portions? Because you can mix and match. Perhaps you want some cheddar cheese on mini burgers, then you can use the table to work out amounts. When buying your meat and fish, check for any additives, many have added sugar or come with added potato starch or wheat. We need one ingredient food here, just pork (although some sausages without wheat or sugar are fine). Read the ingredient labels, every time, you may find you are amazed at what you have been eating.

As you can see, dairy measurements vary greatly in volume compared to your meats and fish, which are quite straight forward. You can have any protein for breakfast but most of us eat 8oz of yoghurt for breakfast. However, you may need breakfast on the go, so this can be a boiled egg (1 egg equals half your meal protein) with some chopped goat's cheese (1.5oz equals the half of your meal protein) and 8oz of apple, for example. This may seem confusing to start with but use your table above and the more detailed food list in the appendix. You will find it soon becomes so easy and it's so worthwhile. There is a more detailed section regarding breakfast below.

NB: Adding seeds to your any one of your three meals is optional but we only have sesame, chia or flaxseed. Men on the program have 50% larger portions or proteins in keeping with food programme guidelines.

SALAD & VEGETABLES

SALAD & VEGETABLES	full portion	half portion	quarter portion
All salad items	8oz	4oz	2oz
All vegetables RAW	8oz	4oz	2oz
Starchy vegetables WHEN COOKED	4oz	2oz	1oz

Fig.4 Salad and Vegetables portions

Like proteins, vegetables and salad can be mixed and matched, for example part courgette and green beans mix, or perhaps greens with mushrooms. However, you can also mix and match your vegetable and salad portions. Perhaps just 4oz salad with 12oz of brussels sprouts. The point is that the combined weight of your salad and veg should make 16oz. While this might seem like a lot, you'll be amazed how much you enjoy eating it.

I typically have a 6oz salad and 10oz of green beans, or in the winter I do away with salad altogether and just have a big plate of steaming hot vegetables with a slab of butter on them! Delicious.

You will note from the above table that the 'starchy vegetables cooked' is a smaller portion. It's not a typo, as some of these vegetables, when cooked are more starchy (but filling) so we have a smaller portion of them. The list is below.

Starchy Vegetables cooked
- Carrots
- Beetroot
- Onions
- Butternut squash (all types)
- Swede
- Pumpkin

Therefore, in the winter I quite often simply have my protein with 8oz of butternut squash, steaming hot from the oven, slathered in 1oz of butter and a little salt. Sublime (for me). However, I have another friend who doesn't indulge in the cooked starchy veg, sticking instead to her larger portions of salad and non-starchy veg. You could have perhaps 8oz salad with 4oz cooked carrots (as a starchy veg from the above list – it is a half portion when cooked). You could have a combined mix of 8oz sauteed mushrooms and onions. The choice is completely yours; the end result is the same whichever route you chose.

FAT

The 1oz of fat you add to your plate can be butter (lovely on hot vegetables) oil, tahini, or mayonnaise, whatever fat works for you. Check mayonnaise for added sugar. It is very easy to make you own too. As stated, a small amount of oil (1tsp) can be added for cooking your food and not be counted.

How we use dairy measurements and variables

Although clearly a protein, diary measurements are more varied than other protein measurements. For example, hard cheese such as cheddar or gouda are a 2oz measurement, whereas white cheese (feta, cottage etc.) is 3oz. Milk is a 16oz measurement, yoghurt is 8oz. Like all other food categories you can mix and match. Let's look at how we include diary in lunch and dinner with examples.

Lunch or dinner:

- 3oz Goats cheese
- 8oz Cooked Mixed Mediterranean vegetables (contains cooked onion)
- 1oz mayonnaise

This is such an easy and nutritious meal because I buy preprepared mix veg (available from most supermarkets, fresh or frozen, but fresh is best). Measure out your cheese and top your med veg with it, add maybe some paprika if you are partial, or herbs and roast this as instructed on the packet. Usually about 20 mins. Weigh your cheese raw as you cannot weigh it once cooked and mixed with the veg. We accept this, and weigh it only once, precooked because we have to. The cheese will be golden and veg sumptuous, and you can also sprinkle up to 0.5oz (15g) of sesame seeds on top of this.

Our protein portion of eggs is two per meal. However, you could mix this with other protein. For example:

- 1 egg (half portion)
- 1oz bacon (quarter portion)
- 0.5 oz cheddar cheese (quarter portion)
- 8oz mushrooms, tomato, onion mix

Dairy at breakfast time

We have one portion of protein at breakfast. This can be any protein but most of us opt for dairy, rather than 4oz of chicken, but if you choose that, it is your prerogative. Meanwhile let's look at typical breakfasts.

Breakfast
- 8oz fruit (use the list in appendix)
- 8oz full fat Greek yoghurt

We always have 8oz of fruit for breakfast, but you'd be amazed how varied and creative you can be with fruit. I love baked fruit in the winter. This can be batch cooked and reheated in the microwave as it is not practical for most of us to bake apples every morning. If you can, I applaud and envy you in equal measure.

Most of us love some milk for our tea and coffee in the morning and there is a 2oz allowance for it. However, this is not enough for some people, so you can take some dairy protein allowance from your yoghurt. For example, if you reduce your yoghurt from 8oz to 7oz – you can put the deficient towards your milk allowance. Because milk allowance (16oz) is double yoghurt allowance (8oz) when you deduct 1oz of yoghurt – you can add 2oz of milk to your already included 2oz. Your breakfast measurements would now look like this:

- 8oz fruit
- 4oz milk
- 7oz Greek yoghurt
- 0.5oz sesame seeds (optional)

However, for week one we keep the plan as simple as possible while we get used to weighing and measuring all our food.

NB: Please note nut milk (except soya) is not on the plan, just dairy milk.

I hope that makes sense. With the Greek yoghurt you can have whichever fat percentage you chose (2%, 5%, full fat) but that doesn't affect the portion size, it stays the same. We avoid fat free yoghurts however, because they contain nothing helpful and usually have hidden sugar and are higher in carbohydrates.

Beautiful Breakfasts everyday

Naturally we do not have sweetened fruit yoghurts. But you can use sweeteners such as Stevia, the most natural and least harmful one (I was told – I know very little about sweeteners, but I believe some can be quite carb heavy. Do your own research if interested). You can then mix the fruit in to the yoghurt and add a little sweetener if inclined. I never bother to do this as 8oz of Bramley apples cooked with cinnamon and some cloves with delicious Greek yoghurt on top, needs no improvement. A few more variables below for you:

- 8oz cooked stewed peaches and plums
- 6oz milk
- 6oz Greek yoghurt

Other protein is available to you if don't want dairy. You might like ham or bacon for breakfast but just be clear on your measurements.

- 8oz melon
- 1oz bacon (quarter portion)
- 1 egg (half portion)
- 6oz milk (quarter portion + 2oz allowance)

I hope that is clear enough, although I do understand how it can appear confusing. Use the tables above and the appendix in the back and keep it simple until you've got the hang of this. We can be more adventurous with breakfasts and other meals later and there are some ideas for abstinent breakfasts to take travelling on the road, and even on planes.

As a rule, your portion of fruit is always 8oz. However, you could also have one piece of fruit instead of weighing it, but make sure it's a big piece, or have two small pieces. This includes apples, oranges, satsumas. But not all fruits are included in the Weight Loss phase, please check the list in the appendix.

This is the bones of the food program which will offer complete freedom and peace around food if you follow it correctly. The side effect is rapid weight loss. Decide on your ideal weight in advance, so you know when to progress on to Management. This is important because once you start to introduce more foods and variables, it is quite likely you will cease to lose weight. So do not progress until you feel content with your size.

A note for vegetarians and vegans

There are many vegetarians and vegans who are on this plan. Vegetarians of course will indulge in plenty of the dairy products and there are vegan friendly dairy alternatives too. Edamame beans and soya beans are going to be a natural stable of the vegan abstinence and all its derivatives such as tofu, soybean sprouts, soy milk, soybean paste, tempeh, miso and any other I don't know about.

You can also use soyabean flour to make food such as pancakes or muffins. Recipes in the compendium cookbook to follow the publication of this food program. You will get enough protein on this plan and there are protein heavy vegetables which can be added to your food. Asparagus, broccoli, brussels sprouts and kale to name a few. I am reliably informed that there are Linda McCartney food products that are also compliant with this food plan. Get creative with sauces and spices and no doubt you'll have as much success and enjoyment on the plan as the rest of us.

What we do not eat during weight loss-guidelines

- Nuts are not part of the program, and that includes nut milk, with the exception of soya. Soya is classed as a protein.
- There are a range of high-sugar fruits we do not eat during Weight Loss to include bananas, grapes, mangos and cherries.
- Check labels, if sugar in any form is listed with in the first 4 ingredients, don't have the item. This might be in bacon, ham, salad dressings, canned vegetables, tinned fruit, even some spice mixes.

Happily, Hellman's mayonnaise lists sugar 5th to make life easier.

- Canned items can be eaten and are great to store for emergencies (like if you burn your veg or protein for example) but check for any sugar, grain or starch additives. It is best to have it in water where possible. Tinned fruit is OK too in fruit juice, but don't drink the juice, it goes without saying.

- We do not have dried fruits, no sultanas or raisins but we can have dried prunes if we soak them for 24 hours in water beforehand. We can also have them if tinned in juice or water.

- We do not eat legumes such as chickpeas, lentils etc… as these are high in starch and can trigger cravings. This also includes humous or any other legume ingredients. However, you can have tahini as a fat on your plate.

- No cream or cream cheese.

- Alcohol contains sugar. There is a growing movement of people who choose not to drink because it offers nothing but a fuzzy head and toxic, empty calories.

- Seeds – with the exception of flaxseeds, chia seeds and sesame seeds (0.5 can be added per meal)

- Lastly no avocado, peas or sweetcorn.

- General rule is, if it's not on the food plan list in the appendix, it's not on the food plan.

Surviving Week One:

Congratulations you've made it past week one. You've done a lot of chopping, shopping, cooking, weighing, measuring and while it's a lot, you hopefully feel so great to be tackling the food that it is all worth it. I promise you this gets easier as you find what works for you. I barely think about it anymore, it becomes second nature to plan, prepare, cook. As you continue on Weight Loss, stick with this food plan and you can add the below to each meal, if you choose.

You can add:

- 2oz of tomato product

Tomato product can be marinara sauce, passata, tomato puree, raw sliced tomato, or cooked tomatoes. Add to salads or use it for cooking, up to you. Any tomato product that has no added sugar, grain or starch is fine for every meal. I use my own recipe to make a kind of ketchup. I'll include it in the recipe book to follow.

To Conclude:

In this chapter we have added much detail about the food plan, without, I hope, descending into tedium. There is a lot to take in but once you get started, you'll soon be flying and feeling great. While the detailed structure may feel overwhelming at first, it becomes second nature with time, offering not only rapid weight loss but also a peaceful relationship with food. The general rule for the Weight Loss phase is to keep it simple. Once you settle into this routine, you'll experience a newfound freedom from overeating and a strong sense of accomplishment.

Chapter 7

Now that You're Slim & Sugar-free for Life

Weight Management

If you've reached your ideal weight, you now have fully realised the effect food, in particular sugar, grains and starches have had on your body. You have a new lease of life, and you do not want to let it go. For this reason, the weight management plan does not change too much, but does allow for more flexibility with the quantities on your plate.

For example, we still weigh and measure three meals a day, nothing in between, but moving forward making sure you have had **enough** salad and vegetables is the main purpose of weighing and measuring rather than ensuring you achieve exactly the right portion sizes of each food group. It is all too easy to under-do your portion size when not paying attention, however, the rigid, absolute adherence to those measurements can now be relaxed. Why? Because a little over with protein or veg, or a little under, is not going to impact your weight, your mental clarity, or your abstinence enough to warrant concern. As a guide, we still use 1oz of fat for lunch and dinner but worry less if eating out at this stage regarding fat content.

Changing up your Food Plan

Cautiously, increasing your protein by up to 2oz at lunch and dinner, to make 6oz is unlikely to cause weight gain, and if it's occasionally under, less cause for concern. In other words, as before, the rigid adherence to the numbers is not necessary. The point is, be mindful but relaxed and keep an eye on your weight. If it starts to creep up, you will want to go back to due diligence in weighing and measuring. A pound or two fluctuation over the course of the month (try not to weigh yourself more than that – we can get obsessive about these things) is perfectly normal and everyone who has tried eating this way, providing the sugar, grains and starches are avoided, have always kept the weight off.

What Else is New?

Another change here is the inclusion of more types of fruit, otherwise avoided in weight loss such as mangos, bananas and grapes. Having the occasional avocado, if you've missed these, is also not an issue. Full details are on the weight management food plan in the appendix. If for whatever reason you cannot weigh your breakfast fruit, it is fine to have just one piece of fruit rather than weigh an 8oz portion. Do make it a large piece of fruit or have two small / medium pieces. This is especially useful when travelling and there are more handy hacks regarding travelling in the next chapter.

Once we have maintained our weight with minor fluctuations for at least six months, we are ready to live a life free from obesity, obsession and the attendant misery. Let's have a look at the Lifestyle Phase.

Maintaining your new way of Life

Lifestyle Phase

You've learnt to live with food, love the body you're in, and adapted to take this food program wherever you go. We've found other ways of dealing with difficult feelings, or difficult people, or just 'difficult life' in general and at this point, weighing and measuring becomes much less important because, having done it a few hundred times, you know your portions and the need to pile up with the good stuff and avoid the bad. However, do not do away with your digital scale, I still feel it is reassuring to know exactly how much fruit and yoghurt I am eating for breakfast for example. This is part habit, but I also know I am greedy and want more than is due to me, so I stay diligent and recommend you do the same.

Little Grain or a Smidgeon of Starch?

But now is the time you can experiment a little more with what works for you. Whereas we had to thoroughly clean our systems of all sugar, grain and starch initially, including in any sauces or gravies, both at home and when eating out, now, with a few caveats, we can try being more flexible. For example, many of us have had success in allowing for some flour in sauces when eaten with large enough quantities of vegetables and protein at mealtimes. This is particularly useful if eating out, or with friends and family. Others are able to substitute some salad or vegetable portion for a piece of fruit after their meal without consequences. Or to just add some fruit after dinner or lunch.

Do not...Let Them Eat Cake

However, a word of caution; we now know, and have established, that sugar and refined carbs are basically as addictive and as pointless nutritionally as cocaine. That will never change. When I look at a slice of cake or a bar of chocolate now, I know I am looking at me as over 200lbs, no exception so I choose not to go there. I stay as diligent towards these substances today, as I did on day one of the program. I know the power they wield from bitter experience.

To quote you from the *Twelve Steps and Twelve Traditions of Greysheeters Anonymous*, "The problem for the compulsive overeater, food addict or under-eater is a physical craving that starts once the person has had **the first bite**. The emotional, non-rational brain is triggered, and the [otherwise] rational mind of the [person] is transformed into one characterised by obsessive thinking and compulsive behaviour." The above is a direct quote from the chapter titled 'The Doctor's Experience', written by Dr. Vera Tarman, the Medical Director "of a major treatment centre in Toronto".

Always keep this in mind when dealing with sugar and other refined carbs as you consider expanding your food program. **Just one bite** can cause us problems. No, it won't add pounds initially, but it will kick off a craving, whereby our "non-rational brain is triggered" and the compulsive cycle begins again.

Finding what works for you

I feel very similarly about legumes as I do about sugar. I remember many relapses that were preceded by 4oz of humous on a salad. I won't go there again. You might be different, and might try to reintroduce some lentils or chickpeas, for example. However, if you feel a craving or a 'need' to eat those items again and again, or find irresistible cravings for sweet things shortly afterwards, you are probably allergic to it. It is a matter of acceptance, in order to leave it out for life.

Starchy vegetables such as sweetcorn or peas were also very triggering for me, so I don't eat those at all now. I urge caution for you too, as an 8oz portion of either is certainly likely to cause trouble with insulin levels, but perhaps you could experiment with smaller amounts mixed with other vegetables or salad. That is up to you. I found other starches were less problematic for me, so I reintroduced occasional potatoes for example, mindfully and not too often, without an issue, deducting slightly from my starchy tubers veg portion. I would not, however, have as much as 8oz of potato at one meal and in truth, I feel better, and less bothered about food when I don't eat them at all.

One grain too many – a million not enough

You may find occasional slices of wholegrain bread are OK, when eaten with plenty of proteins (emphasis on occasional here). But if you find yourself wanting to eat it every day, particularly between meals, or find strong sweet cravings follow, then that's your answer. I keep a sliced loaf in the freezer and might have a slice toasted every now and again, but never more than once a week. Grains are triggering for us in certain amounts, and if you can't find a safe level of eating them without it triggering you, then best not to eat it at all. In this phase it is less necessary to scour every label for hidden grains because, in low amounts, when mixed with proteins and vegetables, it tends to e less of an issue but always be cautious.

The suggestion that you can add certain sauces including gravy if consumed with plenty of meat and vegetables is true for most of us, unless you are at the very top end of the carb sensitive spectrum. For some are just too carb-intolerant to find safe levels, and acceptance of that is answer. The saying goes in Overeaters Anonymous; one is too many, and million not enough. Trial and error will show you as long as you stay honest with yourself and proceed with caution. But always be cautious about added sugar. The rule of listed at least fifth, or more on the ingredient list never changes for us.

The mental obsession

The fact is that some of us will be so carb sensitive that any deviation from the foods we eat in the weight loss phase (in other words, any sugar, grains or starch at all) will be problematic. If that is you, you will know because the peace of mind you have so enjoyed these past months will slip away and food thoughts and cravings return. You will find yourself bargaining with your addiction (just this once today – not again this week) or declaring the program a fake that doesn't work for you; a lie you tell yourself to dive right back into the food. I have seen this a lot over the years.

The answer for you is clean food. Clean of all sugar, grain and starch if you wish to remain free. To avoid losing weight, increase portion sizes of protein and fat, but stay reasonable about this too. Ultimately, you will know what to do, if you are ready to defeat your food demon. Remember, no matter what, we need to ensure we are getting plenty of the salad and vegetables due to us on the program. Speaking from experience it can start to seem too much trouble to cook up a pile of cauliflower or courgettes for yourself at lunchtime but miss this step and we are headed for trouble.

What about {anything}?

There will be some foods I haven't heard of, or I have erroneously forgot to list here. Perhaps if that is the case, you can contact me {website URL} to ask about it, but better yet (and doubtless quicker too) do your own research. This only applies to Weight Management and Lifetime Phases; Weight Loss is necessarily inflexible. If it is not on the list, it does not exist. However, if a certain exotic or Asian food I know nothing about takes your fancy, identify where it falls on the sugar, grains and starch spectrum, and follow the above guidance accordingly.

No two of us are alike with what we like to eat. I'm a real meat eater, who loves her hearty starchy tubers but one of my friends on this program is a dyed-in-the-wool vegan who eats tons of pickles and curds (yuk) and soya in its many incantations. You will find what works for you. And you will love your food, as I love mine, but without the obsession. A solution we have all been searching for, for years….

To Conclude:

So, that's it, the whole program. In this chapter we have looked at how we find the way forward to live peacefully with food after weight loss and into old age. It truly is a program for life. We learn how to stay vigilant but enjoy more flexibility and freedom with how and what we eat. Our personally adapted food plans no longer become about how to control our weight, what we can or cannot eat, and instead are about what gives us the greatest amount of peace and serenity when it comes to mealtimes and living in a world geared up to push poison into us at every opportunity. If you're being honest with yourself, you will know you are living a life where food fuels and sustains you but never dominates you. You'll be enjoying the freedom you've been searching for forever.

Chapter 8

Sugar-free Travel, Dining Out & Meal Planning

Taking the plan on the Road

I don't know about you, but I've travelled a lot and never found it easy. I'm a bad traveller and often turned to food to relieve the stress. I don't know if I achieved that, or if I simply gave myself something else to be stressed about. I would take a carrier bag of food on a plane, including crisps, drinks, and chocolate, fearing that I might find myself wanting any of those items and unable to get them. So, the logic went, I would buy them in advance to avoid feeling deprived on the plane. I never thought this through at the time, only in hindsight can I see what I was doing. Logic dictates we can survive a four, eight or even 12-hour plane journey without the need to pile on the cr@p. But like I said, I never thought it through. I shudder to think how delusional I was.

Of course, once chocolate and crisps were about my person, there was no peace for me until I ate them. Then I would arrive at my destination, sugar drunk and

95

groggy. Dishevelled, covered in crumbs and uncomfortable in my own skin. This is not a great way to start a holiday or a family visit! When I began taking my food program on the road, wherever I went, I found so much more freedom. It was easy to **not** succumb to this behaviour and I therefore, always alight at the other end with a sense of ease and comfort. But the golden rule is to prep and plan because you cannot rely on finding what you need to eat at service stations or fast food joints when on the road or indeed when you first arrive. Be prepared – take your own food.

Certain foods lend themselves more readily for packed meals than others. I have an ultra slim ice pack that goes in my little packed lunch cooler. I take a bag of salad, or some raw chunky vegetables. Mini travel sizes of vinegar and oil come with me, small pots of mayonnaise too. Cheese or cold meats are great when on the road. But if you're taking food to the office, then there may well be a microwave so you can easily heat up your proteins and vegetables. When this isn't possible chunky salads and vegetables that can be eaten raw are a great solution. Add your two ounces of cheese and 1oz of fat and you're golden.

Here are a few travel food ideas that may be helpful to you...

- 8oz Greek salad (adding cooked onions instead of raw makes this measure correct) with three ounces of Feta cheese and herbs, it is such a yummy travel food.
- I make my own coleslaw, chunky cabbage, onion and carrots are filling and easily transportable. Add cold meat or two ounces of mature cheese to this, yummy.
- A transportable breakfast instead of yoghurt would be boiled eggs or cheese with 8oz of fruit.
- Also, for breakfast is 8oz of chopped apple with 3oz of goat's cheese. You can add 0.5oz sesame seeds to this. This is great travel option for planes. And can be used for any meal when on Management or Lifestyle Phases.
- A typical lunch I took into the office was 8oz precooked butternut squash, microwaved with two ounces of mature cheese on top, bliss.
- Visit my website {URL to be added} to download my compendium of recipes for free.

Have family – don't travel

That was supposed to be a clever take on 'Have gun – will travel', but I'm not sure it worked. Nevertheless, people are busy. You may be cooking for other family members including picky kids or you may be super busy with your work and so on. We live in hectic times. I don't know anyone who isn't time-poor these days. So, how to cope with all the shopping and chopping? Simple answer is to shop and cook in bulk.

I'll never forget my first abstinent meal. My sponsor told me to go and buy some chicken thighs and bacon and then snip the thighs up small so you can fry it all together quickly, to that add some boiled veg and a salad, as a quick cook lunch. She told me whatever I bought "...to cook it all up." The words, **'cook it all up'** stayed with me. I learnt quick to batch cook and keep leftovers in tubs in the fridge. I also learned that 8oz is a lot of salad, so I added chunky pieces of carrot and tomato to it. Plenty of leafy salad is a good base, try for 2oz of leaves. On that add whatever you like, you don't need me to walk you through salad ingredients. But you'll likely rediscover many you've not bothered with for years.

I love cooked beetroot eaten cold on a salad, but because it's a starchy vegetable (like carrots and onions if you remember from Chapter 6) we only eat a half portion of it. As outlined in the food plan chapter, if starchy vegetables are eaten raw (uncooked), the weight stays at 8oz - like all other veg - but when cooked, a starchy tuber is halved (4oz) even if eaten cold following cooking. If you have cooked onion, beets, swede, squash or carrots, you'll have just 4oz with an added 8oz salad.

This worked for me, it can be prepared in advance. I would give the family whatever they were having – including cooked starchy veg (say carrots). Then add 4oz of the same to my salad with whatever protein we were having. Alternatively, you could ditch the salad altogether and only have cooked starchy vegetables (which naturally enough is an 8oz portion).

Whatever portions you are having, however you chose to divide up your salad and veg, I recommend you cook it all up, and the leftovers go in the fridge for the next meal. I never cook half a squash; I cook it all. I never cook a portion of anything, I batch cook, even if that means eating the same thing for three or four meals. It makes life so much easier. You'll find meals that really work for you and your way life within the program.

These are some meals and methods that worked for me

Most of my veg is roasted. I used to chop and roast my butternut squash until I saw a recipe where the squash was cut in half length ways, rubbed with a little oil, placed directly on the oven grill and baked. So easy, and delicious, one cooked half goes in the fridge for later, the other is weighed and eaten. Aubergines can be cooked the same way. I tried roast sprouts over Christmas and loved them with a little chilli oil and paprika.

I take apples wherever I go, and I find apples and cheese would get me through Armageddon, let alone Ryan Air. I know another food program friend who travelled a lot with her job, and she made little egg muffins (using soya flour). She loved them and there was no problem getting those through security.

You can find bag DIY coleslaw which is nothing more than raw red and white cabbage, julienne carrots and sliced onion. To this I add my mayonnaise portion, a little vinegar or lemon juice and seasoning. As it comes in a packet, this couldn't be quicker or easier. To this I add lightly fried halloumi cheese and 2oz fried cherry tomatoes (your added tomato product serving) and serve with 0.5oz of sesame seeds. I also have it with cooked frankfurters, or corned beef. When travelling I can take a packet of this coleslaw with me as it weighs roughly 8oz and comes with a little pouch of mayonnaise inside. I bring 2oz grated hard cheese in a little container and a travel size balsamic vinegar (in those little plastic bottles you get in boots for your travel toiletries). This is ideal for me, but you will find your own handy hacks.

Another favourite is fresh courgettes dowsed in a little salt and paprika and cooked in the air fryer; they are crunchy yet jammy on the inside and totally delish. I also always have bags of frozen vegetables in the freezer, so running out of veg at mealtimes doesn't happen. Salad is optional, so you can have all vegetable if you prefer, and during the winter I generally do. Aside from the starchy vegetables, I particularly love cooked kale (note that cabbage, greens, in fact all leafy veg is good) but 8oz is a very large portion to plate up.

I love 6oz of cooked mixed garlic mushrooms and onion on top of 4oz of cooked kale, happy days, a perfect meal. Let me help with the measurement here. Because the mushrooms (normally an 8oz portion) are being cooked with onions (a half portion allowance) they are both then measured as the half portion. So the 6oz of mixed onion and mushrooms would be equal to 12oz leaving you with needing just 4oz more which is taken up by the kale. So, you see how adaptive the program can be? It works both ways, you can have all salad if you like, but 16oz of salad is quite a feat.

I also love oven roasted peppers, courgette and onions and originally chopped and cooked my own with a little paprika, but then I saw ready prepared fresh bags of it in the supermarket (most call it Mediterranean veg) and so now, being very lazy, I buy those and cook the whole packet up in one go. Moral of the story is, stock up on plenty of what we eat and keep some frozen fruit and veg, as well as a few tins for emergencies.

In the early days it felt like a lot of shopping, chopping, and cooking, but now it's so easy I don't need to think about it too much. But I do still think about it enough to ensure I have the next few meals in the house. My husband (not a sugar/carb addict) usually joins me in sugar, grain and starch free meals as he loves how it helps him keep in shape, but I keep some oven chips or

Aunt Bessie mash in the freezer for when he is inclined to have some.

A little planning goes a long long way

I know working people who prepare eight salad boxes in advance on a Sunday to get them through the week. I've seen their fridges, so I know it's true. I only prepared enough salad for two days in advance. That is still four salad boxes. For busy working people, batch cooking over days off is a really good idea. Fresh meat, when cooked keeps for at least three days in the fridge and can be reheated later (once). Or you can portion it up and freeze it for when needed. When I was working crazy hours in the city, I put the slow cooker on a timer before I left. Luckily, I like really very well-cooked meat, but it was also lovely to come home to steaming tender meat which I could add a prepared salad too or boil up some veg quickly. It kept me going and kept me abstinent. Again, you'll find what works for you, just be prepared and be willing to give this a good go.

Shopping online makes a world of difference too. I rarely come out of a supermarket with ONLY what I went in there for. I always pick up more stuff. After all, this was my main dealer! Sniffing out the pastries, and in fact I learnt that supermarkets have in house bakeries precisely to ensure the smell of caramelising sugar, fat and flour carries throughout the store, getting you salivating and in the mood for eating – and buying – more than you intended. It boosts their bottom line massively (and their customers' actual bottoms too). Therefore, shopping online is not only quicker, easier, probably cheaper, but much safer for abstinence too. Your chosen online supermarket usually saves your most bought items so repeat shopping is quick and convenient, and that much safer for sugar addicts like us.

Soya flour and Edamame spaghetti

I was a big fan of butternut squash spaghetti when I could get it, and also courgette spaghetti, lovely with added garlic or chilli oil and cheese or fried courgettes, mushroom and onion concoction. Another way is with 3oz sliced goats' cheese on top, then put under the grill to warm, caramelise and brown. But we food addicts are nothing if not inventive with food and some of my friends on the program have come up with fried and baked options of foods adapted for abstinence using soya flour.

Soya is widely consumed by the vegetarians and vegans on the program, with edamame (young soya beans) adapted for some recipes and counted as a protein too. For example, you can buy edamame spaghetti from some health food shops or buy it online. The portion per meal is the same at meat and fish, 4oz. You can have this as bean curd, otherwise know as tofu, or cook the beans whole or cook soya chunks. You can also buy dry roasted soya beans from health food shops, and these are delicious and crunchy and can be added to round up your proteins in a salad, or as part of your breakfast proteins.

However, this also covers soya flour which can be used to make muffins, pancakes, pizza bases and a whole range of food items, but I still caution you to keep it simple in the early days. Some of us food addicts have learnt how to make pizza out of a cauliflower base, and if that is what you want to do, then power on, but I still keep my food the way it was produced to be, rather processed into something else entirely. But this is up to you.

The muffins I referenced earlier are made with:
- 1oz of soya flour (1 unit of protein)
- 1 egg (2 units protein)

- 0.5oz of cheese (1 unit of protein)
- **OR** 1oz of bacon (1 unit of protein).

High days and holidays

One of my friends used to share how she'd felt it was impossible not to have wedding cake to celebrate the special occasion with the bride and groom, until she realised, nobody cared what she ate. Her health and well-being came before anyone else's preconceived ideas of what she should or shouldn't eat. And, with these thoughts come the realisation, you're literally at home right now, with no weddings planned anytime soon. In other words, keep it in the day, or just in the moment. This is a really important point. Don't worry about your upcoming birthday, meal out with friends, summer holiday. When the day comes, you'll have a plan, you'll feel differently because it's a different moment. Always keep your food thoughts in today, what is your food plan today? Tomorrow, next week, next Christmas or summer holiday. We'll deal with it then.

However, these days it's so easy for me to say "no" at parties or any gathering. I don't offer an explanation but simply saying I don't eat sugar is usually enough.

In the past I have somewhat irreverently quipped that I'm allergic to such food – I break out in fat!!! I attended my very best friend's 40th birthday party, held in a lovely Italian restaurant. I called the restaurant beforehand, said I was intolerant to some foods, and could I bring my own (I remember it was smoked salmon, salad and cooked asparagus) they not only were happy to accommodate this but to minimize embarrassment they plated it up for me and served it with everybody else's. Those sitting near me suffered from food envy.

Never be embarrassed or feel awkward about taking care of yourself. My experience is that people are respectful of what you need to do, and many will be quite envious, not only of your abundant plate of delicious food, but your freedom from slavery of high carb food, and your skinny-jeaned figure too. Not many will be prepared to go to the lengths we do, but if they are interested, give them a copy of this book. I have another friend who (bravely I think) went on a 10-day cruise and stayed on plan. She wasn't bothered about the piles of non-abstinent food those around her were binging on, because she has known freedom for a long time, but ensuring she could get the qualities of salad and veg while at sea was nerve-wracking. But she spoke to the kitchen, and they were more than happy to cook up plenty of extra vegetables for her meals and plain salad to which she added her own abstinent dressings. She enjoyed the whole experience.

To Conclude:

Frankly, if you bring meals with you when away from home, plan meals in advance, bulk buy and batch cook, call restaurants (or friends) in advance and sod what anyone else thinks, you can do this plan and take it anywhere, everywhere, forever or just for now. And you'll enjoy yourself all the more for it, feeling completely present for your companions without craning your neck looking for the food. We call it, "Guilt-free eating". Enjoy your food, but better yet, enjoy the event or holiday with a clear head, sparkling eyes and glowing skin (which are the unsung heroes of this food plan). You'll see it ever more clearly among friends and relatives who suffer from sugar / food addiction. Once that plate is in front of them, they zone out, almost glaze over. The food has them, as it had us, in a zombie state.

Now you've come to understand your needs, found freedom in structure, strength in surrender and a life of possibilities maintaining this lifestyle is about preparation, planning and practise. You've discerned what works for you, and how to avoid the pitfalls that once held you captive. There is always a solution to food plan conundrums, and if you find yourself in one you can email me, join our Facebook group or better still join my Food Mastery Program with round the clock support to kick your food issues in to touch once and for all. The following chapters have quick tips and hacks for you, with more food options and recipes in the back.

Chapter 9
Handy Hacks & Top Tips

Wonderful! You've crossed the line of your weight-loss journey, your skinny jeans will still fit you this time next year, and the year after that, IF you take steps to protect your abstinence from sugar and your trigger foods. One thing that has always helped me is remembering where food took me in the past. I think of that one bar of chocolate, just one bar, which I picked up at a petrol station, with the preceding thought being, 'it's only a (whatever sugary item)', and then up my weight goes and I'm back to where I started. Because it'll always only be one sugary item or another, but until they stop going in my tummy, I'll keep gaining fat, being mesmerised by sugar, and feeling miserable. Moral is – there is no such thing as 'just one' for us. There's always – just 'another' one!

1. Think think think

Tip #1, think the food through to the end result. Remember where you've been, how desperate you felt. In other words, think that 'food thought' through to the end. There is no… "just this once" for those of us who are addicts. In time you will feel completely neutral around other people gorging on cakes and sweets and all manner of dessert. You will be able to walk through Selfridges food hall without so much as a glance at the poisonous parcels dressed up as treats. But for now, think the food through to the end, and what you will lose: freedom from cravings, peace of mind and feeling incredible in your ultra slim, healthy body.

2. **Never wing it**

Tip #2 is …Never wing it. If you are eating out always check the menu in advance so you know what you are going to eat when you get there. Be mindful of hidden ingredients and feel free to call the restaurant in advance for clarity of ingredients of on the menu. This is true of all phases but for the weight loss phase you must make sure you have enough food because restaurants will seldom, if ever, serve up enough. You could go for extra side dishes of vegetables or salad, but I found that there was no problem in bringing pots of food to a restaurant. I told them I had food issues (intolerances, or just elective avoidance of sugar, grains and starch) which limited my choice on the menu, so I brought my own vegetables or salad. They were always very happy and respectful about this. We relax around how much oil or fat is used to cook our meal, ensuring it is free from our trigger foods and that the quantities make sense for us is the primary concern. I still bring little bottle of dressing and balsamic vinegar with me whenever I eat out. Because so often restaurant salad dressings are like treacle, yuk!

3. Certain places I never go now

Tip #3, Some things have to go. I've really no business going for afternoon tea in the Ritz for example. (I have never done that, but the point being I avoid a celebration style afternoon tea, when the scones and cakes are the stars of the event). I used to love that kind of thing – not at the Ritz but other lovely hotels and cafes - but I wouldn't enjoy it now. Although I do go for tea in the afternoon all the time, and if my companion indulges in cakes or whatever, it's not a concern. It's more of when the occasion is all about the sugar filled food, that's no fun for me.

Similarly, I don't go to pizza restaurants, unless I've checked they do decent salads or protein dishes, because not all of them do and I don't want to sit there with a sad little side salad while my companions chomp away, everyone feeling awkward. Lastly, Chinese restaurants because the additives are usually insane, although I may learn to cook some Chinese dishes myself. But to be honest, food is just food now, not the massive event I was gagging for day after day, hour after hour. I'm much more neutral around it now, and eat because we need to, rather than dying to.

4. Fail to plan then plan to fail

Tip #4, Plan ahead. Remember the Tupperware I suggested you buy? This is where it comes into its own. A cool bag / backpack is also very handy here. Because the eight-hour car journey to Auntie Linda's on boxing day, with service stations the only option for a pit-stop on the way... need not be a recipe for disaster. Whatever you are doing, wherever you are going, it is fully achievable while staying on your program, with a little planning and foresight. Planning is everything. You risk being left hungry, cranky, and ready to break your own boundaries if you don't have your meal (or meals) with you. The rule is have your food for every meal, plus one to be on the safe side.

5. Sick note days:

Tip #5: Don't skip meals, no matter what. There's never a good reason to do this. I once bit through my tongue after my mouth had been numbed at the dentist. I called my sponsor with a thick tongue and lisped through what had happened. I couldn't eat, I didn't dare chew. The solution? Boil up 8oz of carrots, mash them and add water to make a soup and add 1oz butter and 2oz cheese. Actually, it's delicious and a handy quick lunch when I can't be bothered to do much more. The carrot recipe is also good for colds and flu and even tummy bug days. You can make any kind of soup you like, cauliflower with cheese, mushroom with butter, tomato with herbs and melted goat's cheese, mixed vegetable, whatever floats your boat.

6. Importance of label readers and online shopping

Tip#6: Meal planning and shopping tips. Without a doubt, until you find what works for you, and stock up on these items, you'll find planning your meals at least the day before pretty essential. You may be shopping quite frequently or finding fresh items that can keep for days in the fridge. As previously mentioned, I find online shopping is very handy, saving my regular items for swift and convenient check out, and when unsure of any of the ingredients, you can expand on the description online to see exactly what you are eating. Similarly, if you are shopping in person, take your label readers (what I call my glasses for long sightedness). Even if you have great eyesight, you might find you need a magnifying glass because many manufacturers like to make it as difficult as possible to read ingredients. Sugar can be added to food such as bacon and sausages (but happily, you can find sugar and wheat-free sausages) and all manner of junk is added to everyday items. Stay vigilant when shopping and initially check everything, you will be amazed. Above all, be clear about what you are going shopping for in the early days, supermarkets can be very triggering.

7. If it's sugar by any other name, it's still poison

Tips #7 A wolf in sheep's clothing is still a wolf. And the many names given to sugar still make it sugar – which is to say it's a poison to us. There is literally more than 50 names for sugar. I'm sure we're all aware of maltose, dextrose, sucrose (anything ending in 'ose' – is no) as being a form of sugar. Like-wise High-fructose corn syrup (HFCS) which has scandalously been added to food all over the States, as way to consume surplus corn produced by their farmers. Its cheaper and sweeter than sugar and worse still, it disrupts leptin, the hormone responsible for regulating appetite, which in turn leads to overeating. Avoid at all costs.

Other names you might be less familiar with, such as Agave Nectar which has heavenly overtones but it's just sugar derived from the agave plant, despite being listed as a 'natural sweetener'. Hell, heroine comes from a plant too, doesn't make it healthy. And how about cane juice crystals, how harmful can that delightful-sounding ingredient be? Despite sounding wholesome and natural, it's just sugar, with "crystals" downplaying the fact that this is essentially refined sugar extracted from sugarcane. Bottom line is, if in doubt at all, leave it out, as it's just not worth it, but you are!!

8. Emergencies

Tip # 8 Mistakes, mishaps and always learning: I had the subtitle 'emergencies' written with a big flat blank under it for quite some time. Then suddenly I had an event that hadn't happened to me since I've been on the plan but had certainly happened frequently before. I had a 'hypo'. Worse still I was in the supermarket at the time. I tend to feel flushed, palpitations, shaky, lightheaded. How? Why? From where? I'm not immune from making a mistake and I'd taken to warming up my breakfast fruit. I did it during weight loss with precooked Bramley apples. Now I'm on lifestyle, all fruits are OK and so heating up my banana and grapes seemed liked a good idea. I remembered how much liquid there was. This of course was pure grape juice, which happened during the heating process. This must have acted much like pure sugar to my system. In a way it's a good thing. It proves the real cause and effect behind the proposed food plan. What to do? I grabbed some abstinent friendly food, in this instance, plain roasted chicken pieces, an apple and sugar free soda and I went and sat in the car to eat it. I calmed, there was no disaster, but boy did it remind me how horrible hypos are and how grateful I am for this food program.

At home, if there is an incident like you burnt your veg or protein, this is when having backup in the kitchen really helps. If we keep ourselves safe in this way, we get to enjoy our food, our health and our bodies in a way hitherto foreign to us. So, cans of vegetables you can abide (might not love – but will do in an emergency) and frozen food of course are handy stables to get you through an emergency.

If by some mishap or miscommunication you eat some non-abstinent food my advice is to try to balance it out with by grabbing plain protein or vegetables as soon as possible. If 'mishaps' keep happening, you may need to recognise you're not taking care of yourself or not taking the food plan seriously. That's OK, not everyone will. You will when you are sick and tired of being sick and tired.

9. Eyes on your own plate

Tip # 9 Food pushers & socials

What has become clear to me is a lot of people have a lot of opinions about how to eat to lose weight and also on what you are eating. I've noticed a smack in the face often offends so a simple, "no thanks, I'm full," or "It doesn't agree with me," and self-obsessed people will leave you alone. Not everyone will, and I can either tell them I'm a food addict (not a solution for everyone as many questions will follow) but most often I simply say, "I'm off the sugar", or a blunt "I don't eat carbs." That does the trick. Focus on the social aspect of the gathering—connecting with friends, sharing laughs, and enjoying the atmosphere—rather than the food.

What you will notice is the gathering will be much more enjoyable as you will be feeling good in your own skin and focusing on the occasion rather than the food. If you anticipate a lack of suitable options, bring your own food or eat beforehand to stay on track without feeling deprived. Taking care of your health isn't selfish—it's empowering.

10. Carbivores and why carbs count?

Carbohydrates are essential to your body in order for it go about its business creating energy and letting you live, laugh, love. Yes, all of that, and some people feel honour-bound to point this out to you. I've had it happen to me, from well meaning, but astonishingly short-sighted people who have seen me suffer desperately with carb cravings, despite eating only a couple of ounces of grains per day. I cannot be bothered with such conversations these days, but you are almost certainly a nicer person than me. You may choose to point out to these 'well-meaning' people that you DO eat carbohydrates (and that this food plan is far more healthy than your previous one lol).

All food becomes sugar in the body ultimately, or rather glucose, but we all now know that the slower digesting carbohydrates will provide a steady stream of glucose rather than a quick rush of it, and stable insulin levels is what this is all about. Experts (such as those at institutions like Harvard) have pointed out that fruits and vegetables are a great source of carbohydrate. All vegetables have at least some carbohydrates, but some vegetables are higher than others. Furthermore, some of the carbohydrate content in vegetables is fibre, which slows digestion, prevents blood sugar spikes and also helps you stay satiated longer.

Have a look at what else high-carb fruit and vegetables have to offer. Butternut squash has 21.5 grams of carbohydrates, 6.6 grams of which are fiber in an 8oz portion. Beetroot that you can eat either raw or cooked and an 8oz cup has 13 g of carbohydrates and are rich in potassium, calcium, folate, and vitamin A. Carrots are lower in carbs, supplying about 12 grams of carbs and 3.5 grams of fibre per cup (approx. 8oz). Pumpkin has 7.5 grams of carbohydrates and less than a gram of fibre, per cup

Apples vary depending on variety, but an average medium apple contains 20.6 g of carbohydrates. It also provides vitamins A and C, potassium, and fibre. Bananas vary depending on size, but a medium one has 26.9 g of carbohydrate and are also rich in potassium and vitamins A and C. Mangos have 24.8 g of carbohydrates per chopped 8oz cup full. We can eat these once past weight loss or detoxing phases.

NB: Nutritional estimates provided by the United States Department of Agriculture (USDA).

Chapter 10
This is the Beginning: Not the End

Congratulations! You've reached the point where weight loss transforms into lifelong freedom. The truth is this isn't just a food plan—it's a liberation plan. It's a promise you've made to yourself to live free from the clutches of sugar, grains, and starches, which we now understand can be as addictive and destructive as the worst substances out there. While you might experiment with reintroducing certain foods, you've armed yourself with the knowledge and tools to recognise danger zones and steer clear of anything that risks pulling you back into your old fat jeans.

Now what?

I've been advised not to make promises to you for legal reasons. I'm advised not to say you'll lose pounds quickly as incontrovertible truth or that you'll feel better and enjoy freedom from cravings within the first two-days on the program. No, the lawyers say, best not to. So, I won't. But I can keep this about my personal experience and the personal experience of everyone I know who has tried this and have said the same.

How craving melted away after the first full day on the program. How those aches and pains that kept me trapped in a body that felt two decades older, about finding yoga in the first week, as well as a laser like focus to get things done. Without that, this book wouldn't have happened. Not just because I wouldn't have had anything to say about food and diets and doctors and freedom - but because of the laser-like focus this food program gave me.

It meant I could sit at my desk for hours at a time, and not think about what to eat next, or without me nipping in to the kitchen every half hour. In fact, I didn't think about food until my husband would come into my office holding his tummy and declare he is starving. We live in a traditional household, and I brook no discussion about that. He takes care of the cars, the finances and the forms and I take care of the cats and the kids and cooking. And we are happy with that.

Phantom hunger

In AA literature it states, "We drank to dream still greater dreams." That resonates with me. I ate to celebrate, I ate to commiserate, to reward and indeed to punish. I ate to distract myself, to help me concentrate, because I was bored, or restless, or worried. You get the idea. With this plan, those impulses should dissolve, hunger be banished and as previously explained, a new freedom is found. However, we are not cured, and while your food, appetite and cravings are in a far, far better place, these thoughts or feelings might still arise, masquerading as hunger. Ask yourself if it's possible you can be hungry and if you're sure its legit, an early lunch or dinner is not the end of the world.

Otherwise, we call it a spiritual malady, the hole in the soul you are trying to fill. You could try prayer (doesn't have to be to God) it could be the universe, or the great creator, or mother nature, your guardian angels, your ancestors, whatever floats your boat. Consciously asking for the feeling to be removed, works. Drink plenty of water and go prepare your abstinent meal.

Your body will know freedom from craving, but our minds are apt to forget how troublesome cravings are, and start thinking, "just this once". Watch those food thoughts, once is never usually enough for us. There is always another "just this once" later on. Where does that lead? The Big Book of Alcoholics, also states that once an alcoholic, always an alcoholic, "we like the man who has lost his legs, we cannot grow new ones." The same is true for food addicts, like it or not. My sugars and carbs 'in moderation' button is forever not working, and finally acceptance of that fact is no longer out of reach.

The End of the Beginning

So! You've reached the end of this book, but for you, it's only the beginning—a new chapter in life where health, freedom, and confidence take centre stage. What's on offer here is so much more than a weight-loss solution; it's a lifetime of feeling fabulous in your own skin, sliding into your favourite outfits effortlessly, and taking this food plan well into your forties, fifties, and beyond. You lose the weight and keep it off without any need for apps, or shakes, or brutal exercise! This is not another restrictive diet with a looming expiry date. Diets are temporary, miserable, and often counterproductive. Instead, this is a sustainable, empowering approach to food and health that works with your body's biology, not against it. I was well into the menopause when I started it and dropped pounds in the first month!

Now I'm on the Lifestyle Phase and have happily got through another Christmas with no issue, delightfully slipping into my tight Levis in the first week of January. Like me you will learn your triggers, and which foods work for you and which lead to cravings. By sticking to what you've built—avoiding sugar, grains, and starch where needed, and experimenting cautiously—you can maintain your weight and clarity without obsessing. Gone are the days of constant cravings, deprivation, and emotional battles with food as you'll enjoy meals without guilt and truly live in the body you've worked so hard to achieve.

One last point I'd like to make

Look, I'm not going to be some kind influencer who wades out of the Mediterranean Sea looking all bronzed and lovely in a bikini. My husband is the only person who ever gets to see me in a state of undress. And luckily, he still finds me attractive. But I'm pushing 60 now, and twenty years of two stone up, two stone down means my skin is crepe and saggy and I have to make my peace with that.

But you, you in your twenties or thirties, or even forties, that doesn't have to be you. If you want to be able to avoid that crepe skin, if you want to have laser like focus to achieve your dreams, if you'd like to walk out of the Mediterranean Sea, looking toned and bronzed and lovely; as smoking hot as any influencer out there, well you know what to do.

This isn't just about losing weight—it's about gaining a life. A life free of diets, obsession, and regret. A life filled with energy, joy, and peace of mind. And yes, a life where your skinny jeans fit perfectly—forever. The choice is now yours. Will you take what you've learned and embrace this opportunity to live slim, free, and fabulous? The tools are here, the path is clear, and your best self is waiting. Let's make this your Forever self.

Thank you so much for reading this book. It means the world to me that you put your trust in my words and this journey. If it helped you in any way, I'd be so grateful if you left a review—it makes all the difference. It might help us reach more women who need this support, just like you did.

Weight Loss food Item List

PROTEINS

i.   All measurements are cooked - where appropriate. For simplicity 1oz = 30g.

ii. You can mix and match proteins as long at the total is accurate

iii. Men's proteins are 50% increased on below (e.g. 6oz not 4oz)

All Meats			1oz =30g	
	Pork - All types inc.		4oz /	120 g
	Beef		4oz	120 g
	Lamb		4oz	120 g
	Chicken		4oz	120 g
	Tongue		4oz	120 g
	Kidney		4oz	120 g
	Liver		4oz	120 g
	Turkey		4oz	120 g
	Ham		4oz	120 g

All Seafood			
	Fish (salmon/ cod etc)	4oz	120 g
	Shellfish (crab/ oysters/ prawns etc)	4oz	120 g
Other Protein			
	Soya	4oz	120 g
	Edamame	4oz	120 g
Dairy			
	Milk - not skimmed	16oz	480 g
	Greek yoghurt (not zero fat)	8oz	240 g
	Hard cheese (Cheddar / Gouda etc.)	2oz	120 g
	White cheese (feta/ goats/cottage etc)	3oz	90g
	Eggs	2 eggs	

SALAD & VEGETABLES

i. Total measurement of Salad + Veg is 16oz for both lunch and dinner

ii. All of these measurements are the same, either cooked or raw

iii. You can mix and match (e.g. 6oz salad + 10oz veg) (or 16oz veg total)

Artichoke		8oz	240g
Aubergine		8oz	240g
Asparagus		8oz	240g
Bean sprouts		8oz	240g
Broccoli		8oz	240g
Brussel Sprouts		8oz	240g
Cabbage		8oz	240g
Cauliflower		8oz	240g
Celeriac		8oz	240g
Celery		8oz	240g
Chard		8oz	240g
Courgette (all summer squash)		8oz	240g
Cucumber		8oz	240g
Endive		8oz	240g
Green beans		8oz	240g
Leafy Greens		8oz	240g
Leeks		8oz	240g
Lettuce		8oz	240g
Mushrooms		8oz	240g
Okra		8oz	240g
Peppers (all)		8oz	240g

Radishes		8oz	240g
Pickles		8oz	240g
Sauerkraut		8oz	240g
String beans		8oz	240g
Spinach		8oz	240g
Tomato		8oz	240g
Turnip		8oz	240g

STARCHY TUBERS

i. These are half portion sizes when cooked but same 8oz when raw

Beetroot		4oz	120g
Carrots		4oz	120g
Onions		4oz	120g
Pumpkin		4oz	120g
Swede		4oz	120g
Butternut Squash (all winter squash)		4oz	120g

FRUIT

i). Only fruits listed here are included on Weight Loss Y

ii). Have cooked fruit (baked apple etc) but dried not on plan

iii).You can use canned fruit in natural juice, but pour juice away

Apricots		8oz	120g
Apples		8oz	120g
Blackberries		8oz	120g
Blueberries		8oz	120g
Cranberries		8oz	120g
Gooseberries		8oz	120g
Grapefruit		8oz	120g
Lemons / limes		8oz	120g
Oranges / Satsumas		8oz	120g
Melon All types		8oz	120g
Pears		8oz	120g
Pineapple		8oz	120g
Peach		8oz	120g
Plum		8oz	120g
Raspberries		8oz	120g
Rhubarb		8oz	120g
Strawberries		8oz	120g
Tangerine		8oz	120g

Prunes (tinned in apple juice only or dried if soaked in water 24 hours)		8oz	120g

FAT

All oils		1oz	30g
Mayonnaise (sugar free)		1oz	30g
Butter		1oz	30g
Tahini		1oz	30g

COOKING WITH

SOY SAUCE		
WORCESTOR SAUCE		
TOMATO PASTE (sugar free)		
STOCK CUBES		
BALSAMIC VINEGAR		
WINE VINGAR		
ALL HERBS		
ALL SPICES		
GARLIC		

Introducing the 28-Day Challenge!

If what you've read in this book resonates — if you saw yourself in the stories, the struggles, or the science — then you're not alone.

The truth is, reading *about* food freedom is just the beginning.

The next step is to **experience it** — with structure, support, and a proven path.

That's why I created the **Nu:Way 28-Day Challenge**:

Ready to put this into practice?

- ✅ 4 weeks of mindset support
- ✅ A daily guide to help you rewire your habits
- ✅ Complete meal plans and recipes
- ✅ Shopping lists and structure
- ✅ A private community of women walking the same path

✨ *It's everything I wish I'd had decades ago - proven path to food freedom!!!*

◎ Join us here https://www.nuwayoffers.com/

It's time to stop obsessing — and start living.

You're not broken. You just haven't been shown the way. Until now.

The Nu:Way 28-Day Challenge isn't just another diet.
It's a complete reset that tackles what other plans miss
— the real reasons you stay stuck. Over four powerful
weeks, you'll rewire the thoughts that sabotage you,
learn to eat mindfully and peacefully, discover how
sugar and carbs hijack your biology (and how to undo
the damage), and finally address the emotional weight
that no meal plan ever touches. This is science,
structure, and soul — delivered through daily support,
nourishing recipes, and a proven path to food freedom.

For more support and resources connect with me at
nuwayfoodprogram.com, including a gentle step-by-
step challenge to help you break free from sugar and
carb cravings—without the overwhelm

Contact me

Keep in touch

I love to hear from readers and people interested in trying a new way of eating. That is why I developed the Nu:Way Food Program

Find out more here: www.nuwayfoodprogram.com

If you have any questions or feedback you can find me at @nuway_tribe on IG.

If you're interested in trying the food program join our private Facebook community here. It's very active, super supportive and people share their recipes and motivational weight loss.

https://www.facebook.com/groups/631468776074011?locale=en_GB

Follow me on Facebook for great recipes and the latest research in nutrition and weight loss

https://www.facebook.com/nuwayfoodprogram/?locale=en_GB

References

Ahmed, S. H., Guillem, K., & Vandaele, Y. (2013). Sugar addiction: Pushing the drug-sugar analogy to the limit. *Current Opinion in Clinical Nutrition & Metabolic Care, 16*(4), 434–439. https://doi.org/10.1097/MCO.0b013e328361c8b8

Alcoholics Anonymous World Services. (2001). *Alcoholics Anonymous: The story of how many thousands of men and women have recovered from alcoholism* (4th ed.). Alcoholics Anonymous World Services.

Atkins, R. C. (2002). *Dr. Atkins' new diet revolution* (Rev. ed.). Avon Books.

Avena, N. M., Rada, P., & Hoebel, B. G. (2008). Evidence for sugar addiction: Behavioral and neurochemical effects of intermittent, excessive sugar intake. *Neuroscience & Biobehavioral Reviews, 32*(1), 20–39. https://doi.org/10.1016/j.neubiorev.2007.04.019

Beattie, M. (2010). *Make miracles in forty days: Turning what you have into what you want*. Simon & Schuster.

Cancer Research UK. (2022, May 19). *New analysis estimates over 21 million UK adults will be obese by 2040*. https://news.cancerresearchuk.org/2022/05/19/new-analysis-estimates-over-21-million-uk-adults-will-be-obese-by-2040

Centers for Disease Control and Prevention. (2020). *Childhood obesity facts*. https://www.cdc.gov/obesity/data/childhood.html

Cleveland Clinic. (2018, March 12). *Why people diet, lose weight and gain it all back.* https://health.clevelandclinic.org/why-people-diet-lose-weight-and-gain-it-all-back

DiNicolantonio, J. J., O'Keefe, J. H., & Wilson, W. L. (2018). Sugar addiction: Is it real? A narrative review. *British Journal of Sports Medicine, 52*(14), 910–913. https://doi.org/10.1136/bjsports-2017-097971

Dukan, P. (2011). *The Dukan diet: 2 steps to lose the weight, 2 steps to keep it off forever* (M. Wynne, Trans.). Crown Archetype. (Original work published 2000)

End to End Health. (2023). *How lobbyists changed the food pyramid.* End to End Health.

FoodNavigator. (2023, June 28). *When 'low fat' labels do more harm than good* (O. Morrison, Author). https://www.foodnavigator.com/Article/2023/06/28/when-low-fat-labels-do-more-harm-than-good

Gordon, E. L., Ariel-Donges, A. H., Bauman, V., & Merlo, L. J. (2018). What is the evidence for "food addiction?" A systematic review. *Nutrients, 10*(4), 477. https://doi.org/10.3390/nu10040477

Griebeler, M. (2018, March 12). *Why people diet, lose weight and gain it all back.* Cleveland Clinic. https://health.clevelandclinic.org/why-people-diet-lose-weight-and-gain-it-all-back

Greysheeters Anonymous. (n.d.). *Twelve steps and twelve traditions of Greysheeters Anonymous*. Greysheeters Anonymous World Services.

Harcombe, Z. (2016). Designed by the food industry for wealth, not health: The 'Eatwell Guide'. *British Journal of Sports Medicine, 51*(24), 1730–1731. https://doi.org/10.1136/bjsports-2016-096561

Introspective Market Research. (2024). *Weight loss and weight management diet market – Global industry outlook & forecast 2024–2032*. https://introspectivemarketresearch.com/reports/weight-loss-and-weight-management-diet-market

James, W. P. T., & Nelson, M. (1995). Dietary surveillance in the UK: The National Diet and Nutrition Survey. *British Journal of Nutrition, 73*(1), 17–38. https://doi.org/10.1079/BJN19950005

Kearns, C. E., Schmidt, L. A., & Glantz, S. A. (2016). Sugar industry and coronary heart disease research: A historical analysis of internal industry documents. *JAMA Internal Medicine, 176*(11), 1680–1685. https://doi.org/10.1001/jamainternmed.2016.5394

Madsen, H. B., & Ahmed, S. H. (2015). Drug versus sweet reward: Greater attraction to and preference for sweet versus drug cues. *Addiction Biology, 20*(3), 433–444. https://doi.org/10.1111/adb.12134

Mayo Clinic Staff. (n.d.). *Atkins diet: What's behind the claims?* Mayo Clinic. https://www.mayoclinic.org/healthy-lifestyle/weight-loss/in-depth/atkins-diet/art-20048485

McKinsey Global Institute. (2014). *Overcoming obesity: An initial economic analysis*. McKinsey & Company. https://www.mckinsey.com/industries/healthcare/our-insights/how-the-world-could-better-fight-obesity

Moss, M. (2013). *Salt sugar fat: How the food giants hooked us*. Random House. https://www.penguinrandomhouse.com/books/211862/salt-sugar-fat-by-michael-moss/

Nestle, M. (1993). Food lobbies, the food pyramid, and U.S. nutrition policy. *International Journal of Health Services, 23*(3), 483–496. https://doi.org/10.2190/32F2-2PFB-MEG7-8HPU

Nestle, M. (2002). *Food politics: How the food industry influences nutrition and health*. University of California Press. https://www.ucpress.edu/book/9780520235295/food-politics

NHS Inform. (n.d.). *Eatwell Guide: How to eat a healthy, balanced diet*. NHS Scotland. Retrieved May 20, 2025, from https://www.nhsinform.scot/healthy-living/food-and-nutrition/eating-well/eatwell-guide-how-to-eat-a-healthy-balanced-diet

Nutrition Coalition. (n.d.). *The diet-heart hypothesis: A critical look*. Retrieved May 20, 2025, from https://www.nutritioncoalition.org/diet-heart-hypothesis/

Oppenheimer, G. M., & Benrubi, I. D. (2014). McGovern's Senate Select Committee on Nutrition and Human Needs versus the meat industry on the diet-heart question (1976–

1977). *American Journal of Public Health, 104*(1), 59–69. https://doi.org/10.2105/AJPH.2013.301464

Public Health England. (2015). *Carbohydrates and health*. Scientific Advisory Committee on Nutrition (SACN). https://assets.publishing.service.gov.uk/government/uploads/system/uploads/attachment_data/file/464627/SACN_Carbohydrates_and_Health.pdf

Robinson, S. M., O'Dea, K., & Lynch, J. W. (2005). Trends in childhood obesity in the UK: A systematic review. *Public Health, 119*(11), 1132–1137. https://doi.org/10.1016/j.puhe.2005.08.001

Scrinis, G., & Monteiro, C. A. (2018). Ultra-processed foods and the limits of product reformulation. *Public Health Nutrition, 21*(1), 247–252. https://doi.org/10.1017/S1368980017001392

Soep, K. (Producer), & Jacobson, S. (Director). (2014). *Fed Up* [Documentary film]. Atlas Films.

Taubes, G. (2008). *The diet delusion*. Vermilion.

Tarnower, H., & Baker, S. H. (1978). *The complete Scarsdale medical diet*. Bantam Books.

The Ohio State University Wexner Medical Center. (n.d.). *A carb intolerance may be why losing weight is so hard*. Retrieved May 20, 2025, from https://health.osu.edu/wellness/exercise-and-nutrition/carb-intolerance

University of North Carolina Center of Excellence for Eating Disorders. (n.d.). *Statistics*. UNC School of Medicine. https://www.med.unc.edu/psych/eatingdisorders/learn-more/about-eating-disorders/statistics

Wang, G.-J., et al. (2013, June 10). *High sugar intake linked to low dopamine release in insulin resistant patients*. Brookhaven National Laboratory. https://www.bnl.gov/newsroom/news.php?a=111548

World Health Organization. (2003). *Diet, nutrition and the prevention of chronic diseases: Report of a joint WHO/FAO expert consultation* (WHO Technical Report Series No. 916). https://www.who.int/publications/i/item/924120916X

World Health Organization. (2015). *Sugars intake for adults and children*. https://www.who.int/publications/i/item/9789241506216

World Health Organization. (2024). *Obesity and overweight – key facts*. https://www.who.int/news-room/fact-sheets/detail/obesity-and-overweight

World Obesity Federation. (2023). *World Obesity Atlas 2023*. https://www.worldobesity.org/resources/resource-library/world-obesity-atlas-2023